Activities for Older People
in Care Homes

of related interest

How to Make Your Care Home Fun
Simple Activities for People of All Abilities
Kenneth Agar
ISBN 978 1 84310 952 5
eISBN 978 1 84642 881 4

The Activity Year Book
A Week by Week Guide for Use in Elderly Day and Residential Care
Anni Bowden and Nancy Lewthwaite
ISBN 978 1 84310 963 1
eISBN 978 1 84642 889 0

Group and Individual Work with Older People
A Practical Guide to Running Successful Activity-based Programmes
Swee Hong Chia, Julie Heathcote and Jane Marie Hibberd
Illustrated by Andy Hibberd
ISBN 978 1 84905 128 6
eISBN 978 0 85700 317 1

Connecting through Music with People with Dementia
A Guide for Caregivers
Robin Rio
ISBN 978 1 84310 905 1
eISBN 978 1 84642 725 1

Creativity and Communication in Persons with Dementia
A Practical Guide
John Killick and Claire Craig
ISBN 978 1 84905 113 2
eISBN 978 0 85700 301 0

Playfulness and Dementia
A Practice Guide
John Killick
ISBN 978 1 84905 223 8
eISBN 978 0 85700 462 8

Activities for Older People in Care Homes

A Handbook for Successful Activity Planning

Sarah Crockett

Jessica Kingsley *Publishers*
London and Philadelphia

First published in 2013
by Jessica Kingsley Publishers
116 Pentonville Road
London N1 9JB, UK
and
400 Market Street, Suite 400
Philadelphia, PA 19106, USA

www.jkp.com

Library of Congress Cataloging in Publication Data
Crockett, Sarah.
  Activities for older people in care homes : a handbook for successful activity
planning / Sarah Crockett.
    pages cm
  Includes bibliographical references and index.
  ISBN 978-1-84905-429-4 (alk. paper)
  1. Nursing homes--Recreational activities. 2. Older people--Recreation. I. Title.
  RA999.R42C76 2013
  362.2'3--dc23
                              2013012277

British Library Cataloguing in Publication Data
A CIP catalogue record for this book is available from the British Library

ISBN 978 1 84905 429 4
eISBN 978 0 85700 839 8

Printed and bound in Great Britain

G.E.M.
in gratitude

Contents

Acknowledgements

A great number of people had a hand in this book – some of them know it, some of them never will. Some of those people include Nicky, Duncan and many colleagues through the years, who have helped to refine my thinking. Sue Keane and the Dementia Link Working team in Gloucestershire, and the NAPA team, for continually throwing me back into the ocean! Rev. Sarah Jones and Dr Derek Glover for believing I could write a book, and Rachel Menzies and the publishing team at JKP who agreed with them. Pat Scott-Exley for her words of wisdom, and Zöe, Morgan and Alison who listen to me rant about activities when I should be eating dinner, drinking tea, or pretty much anything else! Dr Jo Havenhand for help with illustrations and continual support.

Most of all my thanks, love and gratitude to the many people I have met during my time working in activities provision, who have taught me about life and living it, about how to grow old gracefully (or disgracefully!) and how to enjoy a cup of tea at any hour of the day or night.

Thanks guys.

Preface

This book started life as a guide for an activity resource library I created for a Care Home I worked in. I created a series of boxes filled with resources for different kinds of activities, and wrote a suggestion sheet that went with them to give the carers on the dementia units ideas of what they could do to make people's lives more rewarding.

Going to activities support meetings I began to realise that many people start to do this job without any training or any help. You might be a carer who is asked to start running activities, or someone who feels that maybe there is more to caring than making sure people are 'clean, fed and watered'. You may have been employed by a manager who knows that activities need to happen, but doesn't really know what that might mean.

I started in this job ten years ago, and things have changed enormously in that time. When I started there was no training available, and very few Homes understood how important activity was, or had anyone responsible for looking after this area. Now, the CQC (Care Quality Commission, responsible for regulating, inspecting and reviewing all adult social care services in the public, private and voluntary sectors in England) are looking hard at what activity opportunities are provided in Homes, both NAPA (National Association of Providers of Activities for Older People) and the Orchard Trust (providing Homes, respite, leisure and education for people with learning disabilities) have brilliant training available equivalent to National Vocational Qualification level 2, there are lots of books on the subject, companies are providing specialist resources, and support networks are beginning to be set up – there's even an e-zine! Even with all of this, starting this job can be really lonely, and often quite daunting. I wanted to write about the things I know now, that I wish someone had told me when I started – particularly as I didn't even know what dementia was!

You may have a budget, or have to fund raise for everything; you may have full-time hours, or need to fit activities into your existing role. Your residents and resources will vary hugely – although I have assumed that you probably have a high number of residents with dementia living in your Home.

Hopefully this will give you lots of ideas – some of which would have occurred to you anyway, some of which are weirdly me – and point you towards other resources that are out there.

Most of all I want to wish you good luck! Although this job can be really demanding, it is incredibly rewarding, and great fun. I can't think of anything I'd rather be doing than making my residents smile!

Please note that all the books and information mentioned here are referenced fully in the Resources section at the back, which is divided into sections to match the organisation of the main part of the book.

Introduction

What is activity?

Every moment can be an activity – whether someone is flicking through a magazine, out on a trip, going to the toilet, watching the cat, talking to someone or making a piece of artwork. You can turn periods of inactivity into meaningful moments just by stopping to chat and really listening to what a person has to say.

How is activity different for people with a dementia?

Memory impairment can make it difficult to remember instructions, to start something, or to complete sequences of events – did you know that it takes 27 individual steps to make a cup of coffee?! The best kinds of activities take account of these problems, and do not set people up to fail. This means that the process of being involved is always more important than an end result – spend time talking about colours, textures and knitting, rather than asking someone to knit an Aran jumper!

How can I make activities as positive as possible?

Assess the abilities of the people with whom you want to work – how is this person experiencing dementia? Does he find speaking difficult, or reading? Does she have particular interests that can be followed? Remember that everyone is different – as different as you and your mother! Really think about what this person might enjoy, and at what kind of level. Use available resources. Share your ideas with other staff and document any particular things that you think might work.

Set up 'half-done' activities — leave magazines open, not shut and tidied away. Leave things after a meal and get house-proud residents to tidy up. Unfold laundry or un-pair socks.

Talk about emotions rather than testing memories. Use all five senses — memory and communication may be impaired, but the senses are still a way to make contact with someone.

Be prepared to spend time with individuals just chatting.

Don't be afraid — everyone gets it wrong sometimes — you may say the wrong thing, but at least you tried, and who knows, you may get it right. Be prepared to be a bit brave!

Set up 'kits' to be used with specific people — reminiscence material that works for them, a life story book, a rummage box, a bag of textures to explore.

Activity is more about how you do things than what you do. If you are open and person-centred any moment can become an activity, from getting dressed, making the bed or having a bath to walking down the corridor.

Remember that these are adult people, with a rich and varied life. They may not be able to access their memories, but all their life experience is still part of them and helps to make them who they are. Treating a person with a dementia as a child is not the answer, but being prepared to play, to experience, and to join them in their world just may be!

People with a dementia may have a very short attention span due to their memory impairment, but if you meet them where they are, just for a moment, you will have changed their world.

Please note that throughout this book, to avoid 'they', I have used 'he' and 'she' alternately chapter by chapter.

Part I

The Importance of Activities and How to Get Started

In the world of someone with dementia, a single moment may be an activity. If you are tasked with running activities, there is a lot going on behind the scenes to support these moments. In the following chapters we will look at how to go about setting up and resourcing activity provision – from learning about the people you are going to work with and finding out what types of activity might inspire them, through planning a balanced programme, to recording what you do. We'll look at gaining a basic understanding of dementia and how it affects activity, and how you might need to think differently to engage with people experiencing different types and stages of dementia. I'll try to give you a selection of tools to use when asked to 'fix' someone's behaviour through activity, and we'll also spend some time considering things like risk assessing and budgeting. So if you're ready, let's go!

1

Dementia
The Basics

It's important to have an understanding of what dementia is to give you the best chance of working well with individuals who have to live with the disease. My definitions and explanations would surely make a neurologist weep, but they provide strong mental pictures which can work as a foundation for more detailed knowledge as you learn more in the future.

Dementia is an umbrella term, by which I mean it covers several different diseases put together because they all show similar main symptoms. The main diseases under this umbrella are Alzheimer's disease, vascular dementia, Lewy body disease and Pick's disease, dementia with Parkinson's, dementia with Down's syndrome and Korsakoff's syndrome. The symptoms that all of these diseases have in common are memory loss and disorientation, often coupled with hallucinations, and problems with language. These problems are caused by acquired brain damage, just as someone who has a car crash may suffer damage to their brain. Dementia affects 1 in 20 people over the age of 65, and 1 in 5 people over the age of 80; it is progressive, and terminal – at the moment there is no cure.

All of the different diseases give an individual a different route into dementia, and just as each disease is different, so is each person who experiences the disease.

Alzheimer's is the most common form of dementia, and is named after Alois Alzheimer who discovered it in 1905. With Alzheimer's, the brain is attacked by proteins in plaques and tangles. These build up between the neurons in the brain, so that messages passed from one memory to the next can't get through. Over time the brain becomes so silted up with these proteins that almost no messages get passed on. The curve of our learning, from child to adult, through walking, talking, toilet training, school and life, are eroded more or less in reverse order – so the most recent thing is lost first. This is why people with Alzheimer's may have no recollection of going for a walk this morning, but will be able to tell you in detail about what they did on the day of the Queen's coronation. Eventually the earliest memories are eroded, and a person will need help with all everyday activities.

Vascular dementia begins very differently. It may begin with one large stroke, or a series of smaller ones, and its progress is marked by mini strokes of varying severity, the smallest of which are called TIAs (transient ischaemic attacks). All of these strokes affect the blood supply to the brain, causing neurons to die. The damage is usually local, and can hit any part of the brain in any order. This means that there is no pattern to the disease. People with vascular dementia may be able to remember what they had for lunch, but the place where they remember the words they need to name steak and kidney pie has been destroyed, and they are unable to express what they want to say. If access to a memory is damaged, but the memory itself remains, the brain may be able to find a new way of accessing the information. One lady I know had a stroke that left her unable to put on her CDs in her CD player. She re-learnt this skill, but it took time, and her ability was never as precise as it had been. TIAs usually start to come more frequently, with larger areas of the brain affected. The outcome is the same as for Alzheimer's.

Lewy body disease shares characteristics with both Alzheimer's and Parkinson's. Lewy bodies are tiny round deposits found in the nerve cells, which disrupt the passing of messages within the brain. With this kind of dementia there is a huge change in people's abilities daily or even hourly; they will experience muscular problems that mimic Parkinson's, fainting, falling or having 'funny turns'. Day and night often get turned around, with the individual sleeping easily by day, but struggling to sleep at night, and experiencing vivid, detailed hallucinations. People with this type of dementia react badly to many of the medications usually used with a dementia.

The frontotemporal lobe dementias, such as Pick's disease or motor neurone disease, are caused by damage to the frontal lobe of the brain, responsible for our behaviour and emotional response, and for our language skills. There may initially be little or no memory damage, and it can be particularly distressing for those around an individual to live with, as behaviours may change suddenly and with no obvious reason. One man's account of living with Pick's disease told of how he understood academically how his wife suffered from his inability to relate to her emotionally, but he explained that there was no sadness or pain attached to this – he could not even remember what it might feel like to experience these emotions. Many years ago a lady with frontotemporal damage was found singing to a fellow resident who had died some hours previously; she was completely unaware of any inappropriateness, and experienced no emotion around the death of this lady whom she had known.

As individuals with Down's syndrome live longer, they are increasingly at risk of developing a dementia, and this often goes hand in hand with Parkinson's as well. With any kind of dementia there is a huge chance that the person will also suffer from depression, and this will make any symptoms even worse.

All of this destruction of memory means that beginning or completing a series of actions to perform a task – for example, making coffee – becomes harder and harder as more of the memories needed are lost, and some of the versions the brain comes up with on the journey are often bizarre. It is important to know that people with dementia are not doing things deliberately to annoy you; there is a genuine problem, and they are doing their best with what they have available.

Language and body awareness are also affected – you may see someone put a glass down on what she thinks is the table, and miss by several inches, or someone who always walks into doorframes. This is because they are struggling with body memory. Think about when you last had your hair cut, especially if you had a lot taken off. The first few times you brushed your hair the brush 'fell off' the end of your hair. Although you know you've had your hair cut, your body hasn't learnt the new length yet, and is still operating on the old memory instructions.

To use language accurately, we need to have available to us pictures or definitions as to what the word means. We need to be able to apply this definition to words spoken to us, otherwise it seems like the person talking to us is using gobbledygook! We also need to be able to get into our dictionary to find the words we want to make a sentence. Being unable to access this internal dictionary and struggling with language like this is called aphasia. To hold conversations we need to be able to get at word meanings, but also to be able to hold onto them long enough to understand a whole sentence, and then even longer to create a reply. It's no wonder sometimes we need to wait for the answer to come! Arguing is even harder, as not only do we have to do all of this, we have to be able to remember two points of view, be able to compare them, see how they are different, and then explain why we still believe in our version! So arguing with someone with dementia is a really bad plan. When I talk to my Polish friends I must rein in my mind, speak more slowly and use simpler words and phrases; then I have to wait while this is converted to Polish, understood, a reply composed, translated back to English and then spoken. It doesn't mean my Polish friends are 'stupid' – if anything, it means they are working far harder than I am, and it certainly doesn't stop me wanting to be friends with them! Talking with someone with dementia can be similar.

All of these problems mean that people with dementia rely more on emotions than anything else. Their own emotions will be very near the surface, more vulnerable, and often more volatile. As a result they will pick up on your emotions, and feel whether you are giving your attention, whether you are calm and engaged, or whether you are distracted, irritated or upset. As a carer I experience how the mood of staff on a shift affects the individuals we work with. If we are stressed, our residents quickly pick up this emotion, and the shift tends to be stressful. Go on shift feeling calm and warm, and the individuals around you will pick this up and act accordingly. It works the other way too: there are many times when a resident has reached out to me – hugged me, touched my arm, made the right noises – because she is reacting to my emotional state rather than 'How are you?' 'Oh fine…' As a result of this emotionality it's the doing of an activity and how it is experienced that is important – I may be completely unable to make a finished cake that is ready to eat, but if my emotional experience is one where I am being valued as the one who makes great cakes, has the answers, and has done a fantastic job on this one which we'll eat later and which will taste fabulous, then that's a good activity!

Part of the reason that we see emotions displayed so readily is that among other things we have *learnt* what is 'socially acceptable' and what is not. This memory is another one that is lost. This can be a problem when someone starts saying things in public that you really wish she hadn't, taking her clothes off or picking her nose, but it can also be a blessing. This loss of social inhibitions allows individuals to react in a much more spontaneous and honest way than we have been taught is appropriate. People may be able to appreciate and react to art, music or touch much more openly and fully. One lady was able to tell her daughter that she loved her – something she had spent more than 30 years *not* saying, and that both were glad she could now say.

A word of caution. One member of staff I worked with early in my career believed that the best way to relate to people with dementia was to 'treat them as children'. She corrected their manners, their language and their behaviour in the same way one would correct or discipline a child. Remember that every individual you encounter will have lived a rich and varied life; they have grown up and been treated as an adult and an equal, with respect. Whatever memories go, no one responds well to being 'treated as a child' – many children don't either! No matter what age we perceive ourselves to be, we all want to be treated as equals, and with dignity.

Dementia is a progressive disease; this means that you will meet people who may just have been diagnosed. They may become expert at covering up their lapses in memory and are still able to function well in everyday life. You will also meet people who are right at the end of their journey, usually nursed in bed, and largely unable to respond to you. And you will meet everybody in between.

If you are unsure what the situation is, be guided by the individual – after all, it's their life, and their experience of the disease. Go with it. If a smart-looking 99-year-old is worried that Mum'll be cross 'cos they're late home for tea but they were trying to find the puppy, then that is where reality lies for this person. Trying to drag this person into *your* reality is at best counterproductive, and at worst downright cruel. The person you are talking to has brain damage; you do not. You have the wonderful ability to move into that person's reality, and later to return to your own, so use it!

2

What Are Activities For?

Every human being has certain needs, and in order to feel 'well' these needs have to be met. Activities are aimed at filling these needs – not all in one go, but during the course of a day or a week. Lots of research has been carried out into just how beneficial activities can be – people who are given a balance of activities that appeal to them will be more able to make use of the abilities they have, and to hang on to them for longer. People may have better continence or better bowel regulation, be more motivated, or calmer, their mood will be better, they will be better able to express themselves, they will remain safely mobile for longer, have less pain and fewer periods of ill health. They will be happier and healthier individuals.

There are lots of models showing how our needs affect us – the flower in Figure 2.1 is Tom Kitwood's way of showing our needs, pointing out that everything is held together by love. Maslow talks of a hierarchy of needs, shown in the pyramid of Figure 2.2, and when this is looked at in a Care Home setting, it points out that the 'basic' things we need are provided by the Home and the carers, and the things we need to remain ourselves are provided by doing activities. Figure 2.3 is used by a friend of mine, and is a way of breaking down further how every person (ourselves included) is made up. These are useful tools included to help you think about the different needs people have that we can aim to meet through activity. They are also useful as planning tools – have I managed to provide a range of types of activity that will address lots of different kinds of needs?

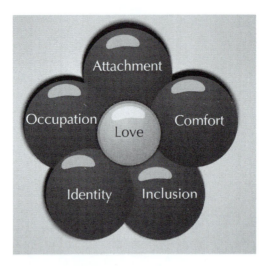

Figure 2.1 Tom Kitwood's expression of basic human needs

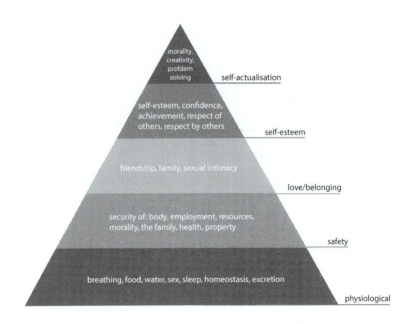

Figure 2.2 Maslow's hierarchy of human needs

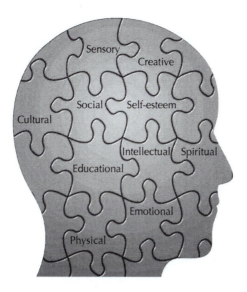

Figure 2.3 The complex person – what makes me *me*?

'If you don't use it, you'll lose it!' one resident I used to know always told me. She was right, and this is the reason that so many Care Homes now have life skills areas, and encourage individuals to get involved in the little day-to-day tasks that have to be done. One lady keeps a carpet sweeper in her room, and after she is encouraged to help make her bed, she runs the sweeper over her floor. It doesn't matter that the cleaners will be in later to vacuum; she is keeping her daily routine, and her pride in herself as a homemaker. On Saturdays after her breakfast we remind her of the day, and go back to her room to change the sheets. It doesn't matter how much she is actually able to 'do'; we prompt her, we share tasks (duvet covers are always tricky things!) and we chat about 'women's work'. A gentleman likes to sit in the nursery corner, singing softly and rocking the cradle with the dolls in. He doesn't nurse them as some residents do, but his son tells us this is what he did when he came home late at night and the children were already in bed. One of his fellow residents likes to help with the drying up, and once started, often cleans the kitchen. We know that we need to go round once she is gone and check where she's tidied things to, and often to rewash the cups, but again, she is encouraged to follow her routine and to continue as she would at home.

This is a great advantage of Care Homes over living at home. We are not related to these people, and there is no pressure on them to get it 'right'. There are many more staff available, we are not trying to cope alone, and we are allowed to go home at the end of our shift. We are also able to meet the people who come to us as they are now – without the need for them to still be the people we once knew. Relatives who continue to care for their loved ones at home do a heroic job in almost impossible circumstances, and often with little support. It is worth remembering this, and the terrible guilt that often goes with 'putting a relative into a Home'. Many relatives like to remain involved in their loved one's care, and activity is one way to do this. A daughter regularly takes her mother off to the kitchen where they work together on familiar recipes they cooked together at home. Some relatives are glad to be included, and as their family member knows them less and less, they are able to visit the group. I have worked with volunteers who helped in various ways when they used to visit their relatives, but who chose to continue coming, even when those relatives died.

3

Getting to Know Your Audience

First things first – you need to know about the people with whom you are going to be working, and what makes them tick. Putting individuals at the centre of what you do means that you are more likely to meet their needs, and create a meaningful experience. Whether you work with clients on a one-on-one basis, or in a group, each is an individual, and each is going to respond to everything in his or her own way. Caring in any capacity is not about a fact-finding audit, however – it's about relationships. In her book, *Person Centred Counselling for People with Dementia*, Danuta Lipinska creates a wonderful image:

> imagine [she suggests] that you arrive at a dinner party only to discover that all the other guests have been briefed about your problems, bad habits, things you cannot do for yourself, your living arrangements, bathing and toileting habits, medical and psychological problems, the kinds of medication you might be taking, financial, social, relational and sexual status, etc. It might be a challenge for those fellow diners, as well as yourself, to engage in a conversation that might actually include a desire on their part to get to know you. (Lipinska 2009, p.76)

I worked in a Home that demanded we assess people within a week of their arrival, and gain a life story within a month. I found this very hard to do, as assessments would need re-writing as soon as I actually began to get to know someone, and a month is a very short time for someone to trust me enough to open up to me. Whilst both of these activities are essential, they need to come after actually meeting a resident, and trying to create a rapport. It is so easy to make assumptions about who people are based on how they look. One lady I knew was tiny, delicate and well turned out. She used a wheelchair and often sat holding a teddy bear. She didn't manage much coherent language, but when she told us what she really wanted out of life, it wasn't what we expected – 'I want sex!'

So hand in hand with meeting an individual, and creating a relationship that gives you the basis to work together over the next however long, you need to be looking at creating an assessment – not just for your own use, but one that gives a jumping-off point for others who want to do activities. If you have been officially tasked with 'doing activities' you may have paperwork already available to you that guides you through this process, but if nothing is available, or if you want to work through this process unofficially to benefit your own working practice, the following suggestions and guidelines may help.

4

How to Assess a Resident for Activities

Any assessment or profiling of a person should go on over a period of time, and be reviewed regularly. However, you may need to make a quick decision about someone's level of abilities for a particular activity. There are lots of ways to assess a person, but one that I like is the PAL activity profile. *The Pool Activity Level (PAL) Instrument for Occupational Profiling* by Jackie Pool gives a full breakdown of how to assess someone, and I would recommend reading it. Simply, she suggests looking at a person's abilities, and placing the person into one of four categories giving a quick view of the level at which an individual will be able to access activity. They are as follows:

- Planned activities: the individual can work to complete a task alone or with some help, and will be able to take part in group work or competitions.

- Exploratory: familiar things are possible, but it is the doing, not the completing, which is important. Tasks need breaking down with one instruction given at a time.

- Sensory: one-step tasks are possible, but it is sensation that is the most important. Things may need to be demonstrated, or written down, rather than spoken. Use the five senses.

- Reflex: the individual is mostly unaware of his or her environment or body. Most responses are automatic, and activity is designed to stimulate the person to raise self-awareness.

You may be able to think immediately of clients who fit neatly into a particular category, some who will need more assessment, or others who may cross boundaries. This system gives one set of helpful guidelines, but it is not the only answer. Be aware when you label someone that as people we don't like being put in boxes, and this kind of assessment is designed purely to help you gauge if you are asking too much or too little of someone when planning an activity. People also like to surprise us, and abilities that have remained hidden or inaccessible may suddenly emerge. A lady I've known for several years had settled in the 'reflex' category; she seemed to have no language, and gave little sign of awareness as staff worked with her in a variety of ways. One Remembrance Day I went round the Home with the poppies, and went to her room. I held one in her line of sight, greeted her by name, and said that I'd brought her a poppy for Remembrance Day. She focused on the poppy, and then said 'Thank you.'

Something else to consider when assessing a resident is that dementias can also be divided into the cortical and sub-cortical. Cortical dementias initially damage the brain on the outside layer where memories of all kinds are stored; Alzheimer's and frontotemporal lobe dementia are both of this type. Sub-cortical damage is to the deeper inner workings of the brain that house the ability to pull things together using memory. Examples of this are dementia with Parkinson's or Huntington's. Lewy body and vascular dementia damage both the cortex and sub-cortex. The reason that this is important is that people who have a cortical dementia will usually be able to engage easily with those around them, spontaneously, even if in a muddled way. However, their level of achieving activity will probably be much less – they have exchanged 'normal life' for life in the moment. Those with sub-cortical damage may not have too much memory damage, but it is the mechanisms of engagement that are most compromised. Someone with Parkinson's, for example, may take a long time to respond to what is needed, but will then usually get the response 'correct' – here it is not the level of activity that needs to be changed, but the way someone is supported to engage. 'Normal interaction' has become supported interaction.

A full assessment of residents should state what level they mostly exhibit, and take into account whether they need supported engagement. It should also detail:

- usual mood and emotions

- physical abilities, including how they get around, and how much assistance they need; manual dexterity (i.e. the strength they have in their hands and arms, and how flexible their fingers are – can they manage a drink alone, can they use scissors easily?)

- any relevant medical history that will affect activity (left-sided stroke with no movement in hand, insulin-controlled diabetic)

- eyesight and hearing

- communication (do they read, use pictures, muddle words, need very simple instructions?); how sociable they are (will group work, one-on-one or a mixture of the two suit them best?)

- other information that will affect activity – 'They love going on the bus but get car sick, so give them travel sick medication'; 'Always has a rest after lunch and will not get up till 3pm.'

Also worth noting is how much residents are in contact with family and friends, and how much *they* might like to be included in activities. A resident's spiritual needs should also be considered (dealt with in more detail later on).

Anything residents, or their family, can tell you about their likes and dislikes – from how they manage their bath time routine (including bath/shower preference) to their favourite television programme – should all be documented. This will help you to build up a picture of the person, and help you to make your time together the best it can be.

A very good (photocopiable) device for recording information can be found in *Care to Communicate: Helping the Older Person with Dementia* by Jennie Powell and Eve Morris. This includes both a life story layout suggestion and the CLIPPER tool (Cardiff Lifestyle

Improvement Profile for People in Extended Residential Care) which gives you space to record details of a person's preferences, and shows you how to make positive changes in that person's daily life. See also www.theactivitydirectorsoffice.com for another template for assessment.

Remember that people change, and you will need to review information on a regular basis (6- or 12-monthly), and when there is a significant change for this person. Keeping records of who attended what will help with this process as you can chart what the resident has or hasn't done since the last review, and how much fulfilment has been gained from the resident being involved.

5

Life Stories

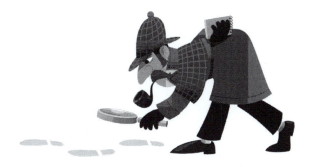

Every client is an individual with a unique story: likes and dislikes; abilities (both mental and physical); lifestyle choices; routine; and current needs. The events, people, information and values encountered are still a part of residents, although they may no longer know why. A person who grew up where people of a particular 'race' were hated or feared (e.g. a Jewish person hating or fearing Germans if they grew up during the Second World War) may react from that information even though it may no longer be appropriate. To understand who a client is, how she may react and what she might enjoy or dislike, it is useful to work on a life story. Some information may have been provided when the client arrived – either by herself or her family – and there are lots of tools available to help us create good life stories. Talk to the individual and her family and friends. Talk to the community, use the internet and look at the person's possessions for clues. If the person used to attend a day centre, contact the centre. Even if an individual is unable to give a clear life story, she will often contribute little stories or bits of information that can be built into a bigger picture. Try keeping a log book for a person, or a shoe box where you can post snippets of information as they are heard, and can be put together at a later date.

It is very important to record all the information you find out about a person, so that others can access it – unless the person or her family particularly asks you not to. Think about who you are recording it for – if it is for other staff, then usually the best place is in a client's notes in a separate section. If it is for the client, why not make a memory book or box? Perhaps a picture that can go on the wall, or a DVD? Use your interests and the client's preferences to make something personal. There are book templates available that might help you. Make sure whatever you make is easy to access and easy to understand. It is the process, however, and not the end product, which is the most important.

There are many things to think about when you tackle a life story. Spend a few moments jotting down the milestones in your own life. Ask a friend to do the same, and then compare notes. Some of your milestones will be positive ones, but others will be bad things that changed or perhaps scarred your life; some people will work in chronological order, while others will jot things down as they occur. There are some common themes that most people will choose to mention, but many others will be individual. Some people may be very happy to talk about their experiences, but others might have real problems with 'traditional' milestones. Themes and problems might include:

- Birth – do they know their birth parents? Did their mum die giving birth? Was there a dramatic story? Where were they born? Do they have a twin?

- School – did they get the education they wanted? Were they forced to leave school early to care for someone or to start work? Were they badly bullied or desperately lonely? Were they sent to boarding school because they were not wanted at home?

- First job – were they called up to serve in the armed forces? Did they hate the job they had to do? Were they given a choice?

- War experience – this has many obvious potential tragedies. Some feel guilty that these were the best years of their life.

- Love – this can also be a subject that covers much tragedy. (My friend's grandmother lost her love in the war, married a man in misplaced gratitude, he then ran off with another man, so that when she met my friend's grandfather she was unable to marry him. The guilt drove her crazy and she would get violent if her family tried to talk of 'love'.)

- Life partners – did they marry or live together? Are they gay? Did they have to pass as straight? Did they have more than one love? Is the person they married their love, or is/ was it someone else? Do they still grieve for this person?

- Children – did they want or not want children? Were they unable to have them? Did they have an illegitimate child they were forced to give up, and does anyone know about it? Did they lose a child? Have adult children become a problem? (One lady I knew was beaten by her son on a regular basis, and was terrified that he might try to visit her.)

Not all life is this tragic, but you can see why taking a 'milestone' approach may cause problems if you have not thought things through. Be sensitive when asking questions, try not to assume what the answer will be, and try not to be thrown by anything an individual tells you – this may be the first time the resident has opened up about an area of her life, and it may be scary! Many of these events may be unknown to family members and friends, and if a resident is unable to tell you coherently about something, you may have to make guesses based on her behaviour. One lady lost an illegitimate baby, was never allowed to grieve for him, and never told her later family about him. As the past became more real she relived his loss and the feelings that went with it. We had to work out what was happening for her, and find a way to bring her peace. Be sensitive when asking family members to speak for their relative – they may find the process just as difficult. One nephew I spoke to had to tell me about his mother's suicide because it was part of his uncle's life.

Another way to approach a life story is to base the journey on emotions – trying to find out what the happiest times of a person's life were, what made the deepest impressions, or when the person felt most valued. Combining the two can be even better! Try to find out what makes a person's spiritual life – it may be religion, or it may be art, nature, music, colour, literature or time alone with her thoughts. This is an important part of the life story that can be overlooked, but the spiritual dimension plays a large part in how we cope with life. Try not to be afraid of sad stories – we want so much to protect the people we work with, but sadness, anger and grief are all part of being human, and our tragedies are as much a part of us as our joy.

If a person is not able to talk about memories, or to access them easily, using old photographs or objects may trigger stories or recognition. Try to make notes of what you discover so that the information can be used again. One gentleman was able to tell anecdotes about his life when I first met him, but eventually lost his speech and moved to a different wing where the nurses didn't know him. We wrote his stories down and put them with pictures from his albums to make a book to introduce him to his new carers. They could read him familiar stories from his own life, which seemed to make him feel calm and safe.

Remember that with a dementia it is usually the oldest memories that are preserved the longest, but even these will disappear with time. Don't be surprised if the recent stories in a life story book that covers everything up to the present moment stop being recognised. One lady's book is titled with her maiden name and the photographs and stories stop when she is in her mid-twenties. We kept the later pages for staff to use, but they are no longer useful for this lady as she has lost this part of herself, and the person in the picture is 'just a woman with a nice smile'.

6

Care Planning Activity

Having learnt about your residents, their likes and dislikes, what makes them tick, and their abilities, the next stage is to plan activities. There are three types of plan that you will need – first, a plan for an individual; second, a plan for the group; and third, the timetable!

If you are tasked with running an activity then individual care planning should be part of your role – the CQC will want to inspect your paperwork when they visit to see how you put 'person-centred' into your plans and then into practice, but it's also a really good thinking tool. No matter how much you love your residents, you cannot hold every detail of a life story, wants and needs in your head for everyone. You will need this documentation for your own benefit. You also need it to show other staff how you can work together for a resident, what *they* can work on with a person, and how to carry out these moments. For an individual's care plan, including activity, what the resident wants out of life is the most important part. Plan for how staff should help individuals get up: 'Alice will want tea before she gets out of bed, loves to chat about her family – which also helps to relax her during personal care – and likes to run a sponge over the sink when you've finished as "cleanliness is next to godliness"!' Then plan for important things to happen during the day. 'It is really important for Jean to get outside for a walk once a day, even if it's raining. If the weather is too bad try looking out of the window and discussing it (she keeps binoculars on her window sill) or take her with you when collecting laundry, etc. from other parts of the building.' 'Donald needs to feel that he is still part of the company he started from scratch. Reading exchange rates and stock prices aloud from the *Financial Times* makes him feel valued.' The CLIPPER tool can help you in this (part of the *Care to Communicate* book – see 'Assessing' on p.183).

Personal care plans are of most value if they are SMART! No, I don't mean that you should always take great care with your handwriting; I mean that they need to be: Specific, Measurable, Achievable, Realistic and Time-sensitive. Look at the examples above. Alice's waking routine is specific (it gives you the details, and why they are important); Jean's day is measurable – she needs to go out every day and it's easy to record whether this happened; Alice's routine is achievable – she is physically able to wipe the basin, and suggestions are easy to add to the current routine, so it is also realistic. Care plans should be reviewed regularly to see if their outcomes are being achieved, and if they are still relevant and time-sensitive.

One-on-one activity is vitally important, but we achieve a sense of personhood through our interaction with other people. Group work is therefore part of the balance of activity. When planning group activity, people's preferences should tell you what type of activities to plan – if you have ten people in your care, eight of whom love to sing, five of whom love to knit, four of whom love to be outside, and all of whom like to sit and chat over a cup of tea, your programme needs to reflect this. I have seen staff planning an activity programme that *they* would like to do, which only appeals to a section of the group, meaning that these individuals receive lots of activity time while others receive little or nothing. Obviously you have your strengths and weaknesses and your own interests (try filling in a care plan for yourself and see what it looks like), and part of your role is to give freely of your talents, but you need to recognise your usual limits and make sure that you are prepared to step beyond them.

Brian Hennell lives with dementia. He and his wife June give talks and presentations on what it means for them and what they want from Brian's carers, now and in the future. He makes the very important point that if you don't know who *you* are, and give *yourself* time and meaningful activities, then you will be unable to do this for those for whom you care.

7

The Value of Timetables

Some planning of activities may have been done for you – a timetable may be in place to give you ideas or particular goals – but it is important that you help plan too – you know the clients you work with, you know what people are likely to be doing, their routines, the times of day that are good or bad. Here are some things to consider:

- There should be a balance of activities – bingo every day would not be good, and it wouldn't meet many needs.

- Planning for resources (including time and people) must be taken into account – an activity needing several staff will not work if timed just when everyone is going on break!

- Advanced planning will be needed for some events – we made Christmas biscuits which needed to be started well in advance to allow time for everyone to make and ice their biscuits, for cellophane bags to be ordered and the biscuits to be packed.

- For clients with dementia a routine will help give stability – a similar event at a similar time of the day and week. At the same time, plans need to be flexible – it just may not be possible at that moment to do what was planned. That's okay, but try and think of something else that might work. Back-up plans are wonderful things!

- Suggestions may be given to you, but don't be afraid to plan something different, especially if what is planned doesn't appeal to your residents.

Think about what resources you will need, and the time and place that would be good; then talk to other staff about what you want to do, or any things or help you might need. Be brave and try it – if it works, then be proud! If not, then talk to people about *why* it didn't work, and decide what you could do, or what needs to happen differently, to make it a success next time!

Different kinds of timetables will suit different situations, or you may wish to use a mix-and-match approach. Planning for the day might mean that you have a display board, blackboard or whiteboard where you can write up day by day what you plan to do. This might take you a few minutes in the morning to think through, and be very flexible. However, it doesn't give you time to find any resources you might need. You may find that planning for a week gives you more flexibility. One timetable I made divided the day into three sections – morning, afternoon and evening – and gave a suggestion for each block of time. You may find that dividing your day up differently, or into smaller time slots, works better. For example, you may choose to break a morning into before and after coffee. For some, this may feel too formal, and for another timetable I suggested certain types of activity – for example, Wednesdays were cooking days. You could base this on some reminiscence about what particular 'days' were used for (Monday was washday, Tuesday was for ironing, etc.). I then suggested a theme for the week, and we tried to tailor activities to the theme – a week when we focused on animals meant that cooking involved animal-shaped biscuit cutters, but we also made fat balls for the birds.

If you are planning for large events, or for visiting performers, you need to plan further in advance, and may wish to keep a large diary or spreadsheet in which you can keep a note of things. If you want to make Christmas gifts from residents to their families, you may want to write in the diary dates by which certain things must happen, such as last posting dates! The type of planning that you do will probably be dictated by what your job involves, and where you fit in the chain of command. Most Homes now have someone dedicated to organising activities, and they may have responsibility for long-term planning. Talk to them about ideas you have or help you need. They will probably be thrilled that you want to get involved. It may be that there is no person in your Home who just looks after activities, or it may be you! Work out a system that works for you, and remember that the more you write down and share with people, the easier things should be. Everyone will know what is going on, and what you need from them.

Telling residents about your plan is also important, and you need to think about how you can do that. A big display board where you can put up posters or write your daily plan is a good idea. Remember to add pictures if you can, as these may help people to understand. Don't forget to remind people about an activity just before you begin – they may have seen the posters, and looked forward to the event, but may well have forgotten about it by the time it happens. Signpost that you are doing something – music, laughter, smells – all say that there is something going on, and draw people in.

8

Getting People to Join In

Once you have assessed an individual, decided on his level of ability, explored his life history, and formulated some activities that you think he will enjoy, you still need to get him to join in. There can be lots of reasons why someone may not join in – some of which should be respected, and some of which should be challenged. Difficulties might include: getting there (because of physical problems, time of day, other events, e.g. a bath), level (too childish or too hard), leader or other participants (having a dementia doesn't turn you into a saint!), personal interests, medical state, knowledge (not knowing or having forgotten the event is on), fear of failure (this could include someone who knows he used to be good at this but isn't any more, and wants to hide this or not be reminded), or laziness!

Here are some suggestions for getting people to join in:

- 'Could you help?' 'Can you hold this?' 'Do you know how?' 'Can you show us?' 'Your daughter's paid for it.' 'Do sit and watch.' 'Thank you!'

Get friends and relatives involved. Remind people that an activity is about to happen, and take them to it. Remember that actively sitting watching can be a valid activity. Think about how you can tailor an activity so that people with lots of different abilities can join in.

Running a session might not be about getting the whole group involved at the same time – allow people to dip in and out, or run lots of little group or one-on-one sessions to take the activity to the clients.

As an individual's memory suffers more damage, he may find it much harder to concentrate on an activity. If you can spend the time working one-on-one, the session may be more rewarding for both of you. With one group we made the biscuit dough together, but then I cut it into portions and sat with one person at a time to make their biscuits. For some people I took a lump of dough into their room for them, and several people made biscuits in bed. CQC recommend that more activities happen on a one-on-one basis as they see this as more person-centred than a large group where individuals may not get the support they need. If an activity only engages a person for a moment or two, it may still have been a valid experience, and five or ten minutes may be enough at one sitting if the attention span is affected.

Get staff to join in! We are all busy people who have many things to fit into each day, but if you can find time to stop and smile at someone, then you've just found time to do an activity! Busyness is only one thing in the way of helping with an activity. People can be really scared or uncomfortable about doing something new, for which there are no real rules, but there are some things you can do to help others – and yourself. In the same way that we looked at who a client is and what he enjoys, we need to look at ourselves and other members of staff and work out who we are and what we enjoy. It's much easier to do something if you enjoy it anyway! Ask other staff to use their skills to help you, and ask for their advice or input on working with particular clients. Do this by showing how much fun you can have, and how much difference it makes. Don't forget to tell people in advance what you've planned – they may have something in mind too and you could join forces, and if you don't know what's on, it's harder to join in. Always thank people (clients *and* staff) for their input – everyone needs to feel valued!

9

Recording What You've Done

It is important that you keep a record of what you've done. This will provide proof of what you get up to and will justify input of time and money. CQC requires us to have records available for inspection – and families often need proof too! A good record will allow you to see if you are meeting needs in the group and for individuals, and allows for better future planning. Most job descriptions now state that activity is part of everyone's role.

Different kinds of records are useful for different reasons. A chart for a client, with a key that allows you to create an instant record of what that person has been doing and completed every day, gives you a picture of an individual. It is important that you only record things a resident has actually been involved in – writing up Mrs X as having been to singing when she slept through the entire session is not appropriate! However, there are other kinds of records that are also important. If you have done a one-on-one session with someone, it is vital that you write even a brief sentence about this in the client's notes – you were the only one there, and the only one who can say what happened! Make a note of how the individual responded, or any changes in the way someone joins in, her abilities, concentration and mood. This is a useful thing to do after any activity, and if done regularly may show you underlying patterns – for example, Mr Z is always withdrawn and unlikely to engage after a visit from his family. Does he miss them? Is there a problem that happens when they visit?

I have started to create photo records of an activity for each individual – I don't do this every day, only after functions, big events or particular achievements. I create a standard poster, then insert the person's name and photo; this gets printed out and pinned up in the resident's room. Lots of residents enjoy this reminder; one resident told me it makes her feel her contribution is really valued. It also says to families and staff, 'look what this person did!' The only down side is that you have to take a camera everywhere you go, which can be quite intrusive, and it relies on technology which may or may not be available.

Recently we also created a yearbook. Residents chose which photos of all the ones available for the previous year they liked best, and we dropped them into a downloadable book-creating tool, which can be published and as many copies bought as we want (see the Resources section at the end of this book for details of websites).

It is also important to review the activity, not just the person or people who took part. Anyone can do this – staff, clients, or both! Think about what worked well, what was okay, what didn't work, and what could be done to make it even better next time. Think about whether the time of day or length of session was right, whether the level was right, whether any resources you needed were easily available, or if you need to get something else for next time. Think about client reactions. 'Mrs X was withdrawn and didn't want to join in, but by the end she was cheerful and engaged, saying, "What a good afternoon!"' That is a client review and worth recording!

You may also wish to keep an activities log, either for yourself or on your unit: 'I tried this on such and such a day, it was great – do this again!' Or 'This didn't work – perhaps we could try it like this next time.'

All this sounds like a lot of paperwork and thinking time; it is certainly just as possible to drown in paperwork in this role as in any other! Most of the work happens when you set a system up – either because you need to try a couple of options to get it fitting right, or because you have to *think* every time you do something. Don't worry, it does get easier! Just as driving a car or brushing your teeth becomes an automatic process that is often done without conscious thought, once you have taught your mind to review a situation in a particular way, you will find it starts to happen automatically. Give *yourself* a review once in a while just to check that you are still spotting and analysing things, but the skills should stick.

10

Sensory Activity

We have already seen how in the later stages of dementia an individual can work at a sensory or reflex level. In the coming pages many different types of activity are examined, and suggestions made for how to adapt to different abilities of audience. However, working with individuals who are at the end of their dementia and who may appear to have little awareness of themselves, never mind anyone else, can be very challenging. It is hard to gauge if what you are doing is okay by the person, what he wants, or whether he just wishes you would go away. Barbara Pointon MBE lost her husband Malcolm to early onset dementia. He died when he was in his sixties. She pointed out, when I heard her speak, that amongst all the other memories lost is the one that tells us how to smile. Suddenly a lot of things made sense to me, and I stopped needing the residents to reward me for the time I spent with them. However, it can still be really hard.

With people at this stage of their dementia, work through the five senses. If you possibly can, work with family and friends, or make plans before an individual reaches this stage. Try to list tastes that are enjoyed, smells that elicit strong emotional memories, favourite kinds of music or sound, favourite colours and textures. Try to use these when you spend time with an individual. Also try to find out what gives the person their spiritual energy and try to find a way to give this input. (See Box 10.1.)

Box 10.1 Example of working through the five senses

My enjoyed sensory input

- Taste: candy floss (cotton candy), hot chocolate with Disaronno (Italian liqueur), fried onions, stuffing, cranberry and tonic.

- Smells: carbolic soap, grass cuttings, fried onions, hot tarmac (asphalt) after rain, grapefruit, leather.

- Music: old-time American, trad jazz, cheerful hymns, lawnmower, children playing, cat purring.

- Colours: green and silver.

- Textures: fur, warm sand, damp soil. Other touch: hold hands (not when hot), hugs from someone I like, hand cradling my head.

A sensory activities programme for me

- Taste: candy floss dissolves easily, so some to eat; hot chocolate or cranberry and tonic to drink. Can we get some stuffing liquidised next roast day?

- Smells: use carbolic soap when bathing, bring in grass cuttings next time lawn is mown, bring plate of fried onions – may stimulate appetite? Use grapefruit hand cream for sensory massage, bring in leather – perhaps toy? Occasional pleasure rather than daily?

- Music: all of these can be provided on a CD with imagination. Bring a cat in? Encourage school children to do concert in earshot? Sing together, bring in guitar?

- Colours: create hanging to go next to bed or round cot sides – include fur and leather?

- Textures: need a cat! Fur offcuts – fake or real? Tray of warm sand to press hands in. Bring in seeds for planting, use soil for texture first, then talk through planting and keep plant in room? Hold hands (if not too hot), hugs unless bad reaction, and once rapport built. Cradle head in hands.

Whilst a resident who is earlier in his dementia will enjoy a long chat, a walk round the garden, a meal and then a game of cards, someone who is in the later stages often needs lots of sleep to allow his brain to process what goes on when he is awake. He may only want or need small interactions where one thing happens. It may work best to pop in every time you are passing and hold hands for a moment. Don't dismiss these interactions – consider the butterfly technique by David Sheard of Dementia Care Matters (for his website see the Resources section at the end of this book).

We talk about needing to take time to allow a person to respond, but *how much* time was brought home to me last Christmas. I noticed a pattern emerging with our residents when Father Christmas went to meet them. Despite all the very obvious clues as to who this was, despite the fact that he introduced himself, and ticked all the boxes for good communication, it took between five and ten minutes on average for the penny to drop. Photographs that I took at first meeting showed blank faces or even fear. Photographs taken five minutes later showed animation, excitement and engagement, and the emotions lasted long after Father Christmas had moved on. If we are unable to wait for a response, then we will only ever get a blank face.

It is very hard for us to exist in the moment for that long. As I sit here typing I am only briefly visiting the present moment – I am also thinking about what I need to do tomorrow, what has happened today, emotionally processing seeing an acquaintance I hadn't seen in years, monitoring what my extremely quarrelsome cats are up to, and keeping one eye on the clock for when the cake needs to come out of the oven. We really are not good at this present moment thing, but people with dementia are streets ahead of us in this skill. One way I have found to help me to achieve being in the present moment is to use quiet breathing and relaxation techniques before and during spending time with someone, helping me to stay with the person for much longer. If you're not sure how to go about this, get hold of relaxation tapes or join a Pilates or Tai Chi class; these will teach you the beginnings of this technique. If this doesn't work for you, try to find something that does.

11

Environment and Reality Orientation

Think about the last time you stayed away overnight in a new place. What did you notice about your room? Can you remember how it felt when you first arrived? We tend to experience our environment on three levels:

- geographical layout: where the toilet is, how to get to a place with food

- emotional or sensory experience of a place: the temperature, and how a place makes us *feel*

- culture of the place: a spa dedicated to wellbeing or an airport dedicated to short-stay customers who are likely to be bored.

The same experience is had by each of our residents in our Care Homes.

Memory problems mean that it's harder to learn the way around a new building, so signposting is really important. There are now many companies that produce signage specifically aimed at residents with dementia (see the Resources section at the end of this book) to help them understand the use of rooms, and to point them in the right direction. There are also other types of signage that can be useful – a red toilet seat or blue toilet water can help orient someone appropriately, painting bedroom doors in different colours, leaving hot food for a few minutes before serving so that smells waft around telling people it's time to eat, or using plates with bright borders so that it's easy to see where the edge is and where the food is. Gesture can also be a great orientation tool – patting a seat so it's easy to see where to sit, or that sitting down is a good idea, or demonstrating an instruction rather than just saying it, also helps keep people up to date with what is happening. Orienting to the space around helps people to stay independent in the care environment when lots of things are no longer in their control.

We all respond emotionally to the space around us. Staying in a hotel I felt no connection to the room I was in, which was both exciting – I was in a new space ready to learn new things on a course – and unnerving – nothing felt homely, I could hear other people through the walls and the lights were too bright. Our five senses and our emotional memory are all part of this experience. If we change the space around us we can change the mood, and our experience – for example, what music is playing, or what programme is on the television, what things are lying around, what we can smell. Creating a positive emotional reaction to a place can help people feel at home even if they are no longer able to remember why they are here or to find their way around.

Part of our role as activity providers is to make a difference to the environment. We may not be able to make big changes – an easy-access garden or a new signage system are beyond our role (although hopefully we can make suggestions and pressure for change) – but changing a person's emotional experience by creating a culture of activity is hopefully something we can all do. An activity culture means that it always feels like there is something going on, or just gone on, or about to happen. Half-done activities are around, people are encouraged to join in with daily tasks such as laying the table, art and craft work is on display, as are photographs of people having a good time, the television and radio are tuned to reflect residents' tastes (or turned off) and staff chat to residents more than to each other, and are able to share meal times. Groups or pairings of people are not exclusive – newcomers are welcomed, smiled at or waved to as they arrive or pass by, although one-on-one communication is respected, and people are allowed to 'just be' if they choose. Some of this we can achieve alone, but other things involve teamwork and management support. If you feel you are alone, make what changes you can to your own way of working, and try to challenge the things that feel like barriers.

As well as being a means of describing how to keep people 'found' in your Home, 'reality orientation' is the name of a communication tool. The idea is that, no matter what, you will correct a person with a dementia worldview to that of the 'real' one. This includes reminding them that a husband or wife is dead, that they are actually in their eighties, that their parents are dead, that they live in a Care Home, or that it's actually Tuesday and time for lunch. Reality orientation has its place, but as our understanding of dementia has progressed, it is (thank goodness) no longer the only communication tool at our disposal. Options include Penny Garner's SPECAL method (see Oliver James' book in the Resources section at the end of this book), which starts with the instruction never to argue with someone with a dementia, and goes on to build an entire strategy for care and communication which begins at diagnosis and lasts far beyond a person moving into care; using reminiscence or validation. Each of these tools has their place, and the best way of showing this I have seen was created by Colin Barnes, a specialist speech and language therapist, in his MA thesis 'Chatter Matters'. Colin suggests that you take a basic pronouncement made by a person with a dementia – for example, 'Wasn't it nice to see Theresa walking the dogs on Tuesday?' – and look at which stage of a dementia this person is experiencing. This will then help you to decide how best to answer that person. (See Figure 11.1.)

Early in a person's experience of dementia they are usually aware of the disease, and are able to appreciate re-orientation. The person may use diaries, lists or other strategies to help in remembering things. With the statement above about dogs, you can be sure that there was a walk, and there were dogs, but maybe the person mis-remembers the day, or the person's name. Correcting them tactfully is a good thing.

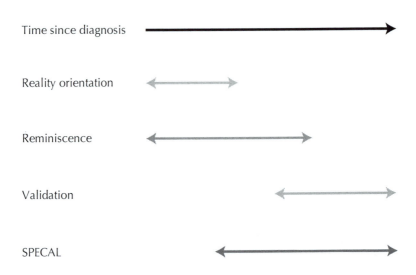

Time since diagnosis

Reality orientation

Reminiscence

Validation

SPECAL

Figure 11.1 Communication strategies
through the stages of dementia

As the dementia progresses, it becomes more important to use reminiscence – usually a good clue is that forcing your own view of the truth causes distress. With the dog example there may or may not have been a walk, but maybe this person is remembering an event from long ago, or reinterpreting an event to make sense of it. Rather than insisting on the truth as you see it, think about what the person is trying to communicate. Ask if she had a dog, or share a story rather than correcting her. You can use this technique either after she has made an 'error' or in anticipation of difficulty. Once distracted, a person can talk about a subject with which she is more familiar.

In validation, clients are encouraged to lead the conversation whilst you mirror their emotions, words, facial expressions and body language to keep them talking. It is likely that there wasn't a walk, but that the person is making sense of an emotion or memory through talking about this supposed incident. Ironically, being listened to can help a person make more sense as she 'connects'. Let her tell you about her ideas. Validation is very quality-focused, although only works when residents have poor insight into their dementia.

Penny Garner's strategy for wraparound care is SPECAL, and I would recommend reading her book to understand how deeply she sees it working (see Oliver James' book in the Resources section at the end of this book). However, her basic rule is *never* to argue with someone who has dementia, which means that, if necessary, you will go along with a person's worldview even if you 'know' it's not true, because it *is* true for the person. For instance, someone who has not been out, or received visitors for some months, and therefore has not been on a walk or seen any dogs, believes that this thing has happened, and you should encourage the person to talk about what took place. This may be challenging for you, but in some situations it may be in both your best interests to do this. This approach can work well with people who imagine they are in a previous role – for example, still at work.

Ultimately your knowledge of your residents will help you make the decision about what type of communication is appropriate. One lady asked repeatedly throughout the day about where her husband was. Some of the carers, not wanting to cause her distress by telling her he was dead, responded instead with helpful suggestions – 'Maybe he's still at work?' 'What's he like – is he very handsome?' This lady would get very distressed because she thought she knew her husband was dead and was asking for reassurance on this point. The carers looked at her level of dementia, and thought they were getting it right, but in this instance, knowledge of the individual was more important.

For a greater understanding of the problems and challenges of communication when you have a dementia read *Care to Communicate* by Jennie Powell and Eve Morris (see 'Assessing', p.183). This book also gives lots of further examples of what makes good and bad communication, and is full of helpful illustrations.

12

Using Activity to 'Solve Problems'

We have already talked about how a person with dementia has suffered brain damage, and can no longer join us in 'our' world. However, in many Care Homes people are labelled as 'wanderers', 'shouters', 'challenging' or 'aggressive' because of the behaviour we observe in them. All too often, as providers of activities, we are asked to 'fix' these 'problems'.

Imagine for a moment that you find yourself in the supermarket. Someone is talking to you, and you're not sure who they are. You can't think how you got here, it's noisy, it's bright, there are people all around you. You might well be overwhelmed by what is going on around you – frightened as to how you got there, unable to make sense of what the person in front of you is trying to tell you, not sure if you know who they are. Or remember the moment when you come out of the cinema in the dark and you suddenly have *no idea* where you parked the car. Think about the emotions you experienced – fear, anger, maybe even panic. These situations, for us, can usually be resolved – we might have had a moment of lapsed concentration and 'come to' in the shop – the dislocation is only momentary. The car is usually found pretty quickly, and if not, most of us have a mobile phone, and someone to ask for help. But imagine if you are unable to wake up from this situation. Or even worse, if these situations played out one after the other, as you try frantically to interpret the world you are presented with by means of memories that are still intact. And into this, add that suddenly someone is taking your trousers down, because they think you should go to the toilet. Perhaps you might lash out? Swear? Refuse to behave *sensibly*? This is the closest we can get to explaining the way some people experience their dementia – for all or part of their journey. If you look at the situation like this, lashing out or shouting are actually pretty reasonable responses to a scary situation. The 'problem' is not the behaviour – that is, part of the person's need to communicate that life is frightening, or too much – but that we cannot see into a person's mind to see what else is going on for him. Indeed, if you follow this to its conclusion, it is often *our* behaviour that is the 'problem' – approaching someone and trying to do something without enough warning, clues or time to understand, doing *to* people, rather than *with* them.

If you are able to approach the behaviour of those who are in your care, bearing in mind that all behaviour is trying to communicate something, this may give you a clue to what the underlying problem is. Only by unpacking a person's behaviour, finding the reasons behind it, can we hope to offer even part of a solution. In his book *And Still the Music Plays: Stories of People with Dementia*, Graham Stokes tells of many such unpackings – from the man who kept collecting everyone on the unit's waste bins, to the lady who couldn't be in her bedroom because it was purple. In many of his examples, it is life story work that is able to provide the key to working out what is behind the behaviour described.

If you are asked to 'solve' someone's behaviour, start by looking at everything around the person. Try keeping a behaviour chart and try to find out what triggers the behaviour – is it time of day, actions of others, particular words or events, noise levels, seeing something? Try to find patterns. Look at the life story, or go back to those people who are able to tell you about a person's history, and explain that you are trying to come up with some possible reasons for the way a relative is behaving. Do they have any clues? Be tactful – this can be a difficult conversation to have, especially if the behaviour you are trying to decode is offensive in any way. Try to involve the whole team in what you are doing.

If you need quick 'fixes', work on what you already know of a person. Use the different communication tools discussed – does someone need you to join them in the 'it's criminal what they're doing to me' club? Mirror behaviour and facial expressions to feed back that you are joining the person where he is. Offer validation, or reassurance. Consider distracting him onto something else – this works best if combined with validation and reassurance. Share people's language – a lady I know swears like a trooper when someone tries to help her with her personal care. I have had quite a lot of success joining her in her world, repeating back to her the words she is using, even though generally there is no way I would consider it appropriate to swear in front of a resident. If your colleagues think you've gone slightly mad, just make sure you explain when you have a minute what you are up to! Try not to explain over someone's head, however – or bang will go all your hard work.

All of these techniques are part of what activity is – it is every moment of daily life, even the bad moments! Once you've identified triggers, or brought someone back from a really bad place, your knowledge of his likes and dislikes around activity can be used to move him into an even better place. Painting calms one gentleman down – especially if classical music is playing in the background. Darning helps another lady to feel as if she is useful, especially if you can share tea and a chat at the same time. Eventually, if you are able to spot the triggers, you can hope to cut straight from the potential trigger – '3pm is always going to be noisy and noise is Mr X's trigger – to the good place – at 2.45pm, take Mr X to a quiet room where he can paint and listen to classical music.'

13

Assessing the Risks

After getting into trouble for bringing unauthorised eggs to a cooking session, I have been very keen on spotting the things that others may consider to be risks – hence some of the suggestions in the pages that follow! For some activities or events there may already be risk assessments completed, and it's just a case of finding them and then following – or challenging – them. Otherwise you need to invent your own.

Basically a risk is something that may or may not cause a problem to or for someone. A risk assessment is designed to spot these problems (hopefully before they occur), and to set in place procedures to control or remove the risk (see Box 13.1).

If in doubt as to whether something could be considered a risk, work through these steps and think of every objection someone could come up with; then, if you are challenged, you should be able to answer appropriately. If you think you've identified something that is a high risk, or about which you are not sure or need advice, *tell someone!* Your Home will already have lots of risk assessments that you should be able to access; there should also be blank forms ready to fill in. I keep copies of any assessments I have completed so that I know what procedures I should follow. This is particularly important around trips out as you may be beyond your usual support network and need to know how you will manage a situation.

Box 13.1 Example of a risk assessment

Use of strong adhesives, for example UHU or Superglue, by residents or by activities staff in presence of residents.

Risk: Inhalation of fumes or ingestion of product may cause illness in residents or staff. Unsupervised or inappropriate use of products may cause harm to residents and staff, or damage to property.

Is risk high, medium or low? Medium.

What systems are already in place to deal with this situation? COSHH (Control of Substances Hazardous to Health) sheets are available for these products. Products are currently used rarely, and use is always supervised.

What can be done to further minimise or remove risks? Products can be replaced by safe glue, for example PVA, which has no fumes and is non-toxic and water-soluble. Any item that will need stronger glue should be passed to the maintenance team, and the products should only be used in the maintenance workshop.

Risk once control measures are in place: Removed.

We want to keep our residents safe, but there is such a thing as wrapping people in too much cotton wool. For example, a lady with dementia may live in a secure unit as she is unable to appreciate personal danger, and believes that she lives in another country in 1920. Such restraint is acceptable. What would not be acceptable would be then preventing that lady from walking around in the secure unit as she is a little unsteady and may fall. If we have identified this lady to be at risk of falls, the situation should be managed to allow her to maintain as much independence as possible – for example, by managing the risk associated with falls by helping her to wear hip protectors, making sure she wears good shoes with well-maintained soles, making sure that the place is free of trip hazards, and discussing with her family the reasoning behind considering that this is an acceptable risk. Don't decide that activities are too risky without good reason.

14

Budgeting and Money Stretching

Here again your role will play a huge part in how much you will have to do with budgeting, as will the Home you work for. Some Homes have a dedicated budget for activities, and some demand that money must be raised by the activities person or team for anything they want to do. Your Home will also have systems in place as to how they want you to be accountable for money. The best person to find out this information from is a Home's administrator.

I am lucky, I have always worked within a budget, and have not yet had to fund raise for my bread and butter. There are many books available that will give you good advice on this – or check out www. better-fundraising-ideas.com. Everybody is short of money at the moment, but even so, you should be able to get a case together for being given a budget – even if it's only very small. This is where recording what you do, and how it affects people, is so important.

If you have a budget you need to be very clear about what it covers – do you have to buy your own stationery items, pay for developing of photographs or for ingredients needed for a cooking session? Are you responsible for replacing large items such as CD or DVD players? Is there money for cups of tea on an outing? If you want something do you need to create a purchase order and get it signed before you are allowed to spend the money?

If you have a budget you need to plan how you are going to spend it, and make sure you record everything so that it is easy to show where the money goes, and what use you make of it. Planning for your budget you need to think about long-term plans – do you want outside speakers or entertainers for a special event? Do you need to buy craft supplies for a particular project? Can you carry forward money from one month to the next?

Making money go further is always a challenge. Think about value – if someone offers to come in and run a session that will cost you £100, is it worth it? Could you get the same for less somewhere else, or use the talents of those around you to do it for free? Could you go on a training course for the same money, and then run hundreds of the session?

Shop in charity shops, flea markets and jumble sales, car boots and on eBay or similar sites for bargains, but make sure it is a bargain before you commit. Keep a list of all the things you would like, want or need, so that you don't get seduced by something that isn't really going to do the job. Keep receipts for everything, and check with your administrator whether it needs to be itemised. Keep a notebook and pen with you and offer them if someone is reluctant to give a receipt. Explain that it's just so you can get your own money back from your place of work. Ask relatives and other staff for help – we made our own hedgerow wine last year, and everyone saved bottles for us; we encouraged everyone to bring in unused china to create a huge tea set with lots of choice about which cup people wanted. If you have good relationships with local schools and businesses, find out if they can offer you sponsorship in kind – leftover paints at the end of term, storage containers that can be turned into craft activities. Find out if there is a local scrapstore or resource centre (see www.scrapstoresuk.org). We have one locally where new items for craft are sold at reduced prices, and local firms donate all kinds of weird and wonderful waste from their own work, which, with a little imagination, can become almost anything!

Try not to get bogged down. Remember how we talked about just smiling at someone being a valuable activity?

15

Trouble

We need to celebrate the good times and the achievements of activities and care staff, but if your personal experience leaves you feeling demoralised, then you need to feel you are not alone! A member of the care staff working with me late in her pregnancy turned to me at the end of her first week and said, 'I can see why you're always in trouble!' She went on to explain that activities was so much more freelance than care, and that we related to the residents as friends, so were 'on their side' rather than on that of 'The Firm'. Although it started to sound like a bad gangster movie, I knew what she meant. I don't wear a uniform, so my relationship with our residents *is* different. I don't invade their physical privacy, I take them out, I want to know about their lives, and I give them time to express themselves. I try to become 'one of them'. I see that as what I am employed to do. The thing is that this is not how everyone else sees my role, and this is usually why I'm often 'in trouble'!

Sometimes there is no help for this — a member of a domestic team I worked with explained once that the only activities she saw as real activity were the big functions, so that when I worked with small groups or individuals, I was wasting everyone's time. I can see what she meant — with dozens of people to work with, how could I justify spending time with just one? I've been labelled 'lazy' for sitting having a conversation with someone, and told that my job is a 'doss job'. This has much more to do with the people who handed out these comments than with me. If you are genuinely doing all you can for your residents without giving too much time to those you naturally get along with better, and if you are creating a balance of opportunities, you have to believe in yourself. The best thing to do about this kind of 'trouble' is to mention things to someone in higher authority – perhaps a training manager if you have one. Every one of the members of the staff team, be they domestic, kitchen, administration, maintenance, care, management or activities, has a responsibility to work actively with residents. It may be an uphill task, but at some point they are going to need training in this. Have a look at some of the wonderful publications from NAPA (see the Resources section at the end of the book) about how to educate your colleagues.

The other kind of trouble I am most frequently guilty of is not telling the right people about my crazy ideas! We need to have new ideas, to be able to think outside the box, but this doesn't make us easy to work with, or to manage! Talk to people! Talk to your colleagues, talk to those below you in the chain, and consult with (don't *tell*) your line manager and, if it's appropriate, your Home manager. If it's at all possible set up a regular meeting time with management, so that you can run all your new ideas past them for initial problem spotting, then keep them up to date with how things are going.

There are likely to be times when your latest wonderful idea clashes head on with management. This may be because we are not shown the biggest picture of everything that is going on. A soldier may be ordered to a course of action without understanding all the events and pressures that have led to the order being created. He doesn't need to know all this to carry out his job – indeed, knowing may mean that he is unable to carry it out with his whole mind. Sometimes the orders are right, and sometimes they're just daft. You will have to decide for yourself how far you wish to challenge the authorities, and how to go about doing this.

If you feel personally unsafe, but that your course of action is justified, you may like to consider joining a union. There is no one yet who specialises in activities personnel, but using a union finder on the internet may help you find one that fits the bill.

Remember that most trouble comes from lack of communication, so just keep talking!

Part II

But What Can I Actually Do?

Each topic that follows gives you suggestions of what to do with residents of different abilities, with groups and in one-on-one sessions. Look at any timetable that is provided; this may give you suggestions that you just have to carry out. NB: The pages appear in alphabetical order, not in order of importance.

You could join NAPA (National Association for Providers of Activities for Older People), a fabulous organisation. Many Care

Homes are members, but you can join as an individual. They welcome overseas members, send out regular newsletters and inspiration magazines (www.napa-activities.co.uk).

Brainstorm with other staff if you are looking for a solution to a particular problem, or for a particular resource.

There are many internet sites with suggestions of things you can do. Try searching for activities on Google or another search engine, but think about who the suggestions are aimed at. Many early education sites offer suggestions that just need to be tweaked a little before older clients can use them.

There are many books available – try *Keeping Busy* by James R. Dowling for a start!

If you find you are very busy at a particular time, why not load your pockets with two-minute activities – a picture that will evoke an emotion or reminiscence that you can chat with someone about; a tube of bubbles to blow; a small pot of hand cream to rub on someone's hands; balloons that you can blow up, bat around and leave with someone; tactile fabric or wool that a client can enjoy sitting and stroking or untangling; or even a glove puppet! It only takes a moment to change someone's day.

Don't forget that just taking the time to smile at people, to really listen when they talk, is a really valuable activity. By being brave and giving a little of yourself, you will get a lot in return!

Art

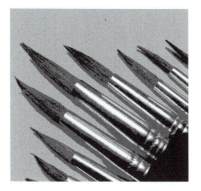

Suggested resources

Felt-tip pens

Watercolour and acrylic paints

Pencil crayons

Pencils

Assorted paintbrushes

Eraser and pencil sharpener

Assorted paper

Colouring sheets

Paint palettes

Books or magazines full of art pictures

Risks

- Hopefully the paints, etc. should be washable – although acrylic will set. If it gets onto clothes, try to wash it off immediately. Any paint that gets onto paintwork or soft furnishings should be wiped off quickly and maintenance or housekeeping staff alerted.

- Be aware of brushes and pens as 'sharp' objects.

Some suggestions

- Some residents will be quite happy to paint from their imagination.

- Provide sources or objects to copy, or colouring sheets for adults for those less able (Winslow® produce 'age-appropriate' colouring sheets – see www.winslowresources.com).

- Be prepared to join in, and be part of the 'I'm no good at art' club!

- Don't worry if individuals paint the table, the floor, themselves or each other! Provide aprons if you are concerned about clothes (disposable ones used in personal care are ideal), and clear the area of table linen, etc.

- Consider using finished art in cards, etc. – many Homes like to use residents' card designs, or send individual ones to families. You could get pieces professionally printed at an online printing service, such as www.vistaprint.co.uk or www.ecoartcards.com in the UK.

- Art therapists work with watercolour paper saturated in water, then brush long sweeps of watercolour paint over it, allowing the colours to mix. Try running a sensory session using this technique (see page 70).

- If residents paint blocks of colour, you could doctor them to make displays – cut things out, mount shapes and make collages, or use a black marker to draw on the page. Get the artist to help you decide what it is you're drawing.

- You could use specialist paints such as glass paints. We did a very successful stained glass project with glass paint pens (*much* less messy than the pot version!) on overhead projector sheets, and clear plastic food bags. We had fun with the colours when painting, then we fixed the dry pieces to the windows and enjoyed the effect of the shadows they created on the floor. NB: If you hang art up to dry, liquid paint will run – although this can create an interesting effect, if it drips onto the floor, it will stain.

- Residents can use ceramic pens to decorate their own mugs – this has the added advantage of encouraging them to use a larger personalised mug for drinks, giving them a larger fluid intake. The mugs will need heat fixing before washing, otherwise you will lose the artwork. For individuals with weak wrists, or who need plastic beakers, use the glass paint pens.

- Pastels – the soft kind, not the oil-based kind – are great for sensory art as you need little pressure to make a mark, and the colours are fully blendable. You will need a fixative spray to keep the art from deteriorating, or you could laminate the finished products and use them as tablemats, etc.

- Do finger painting! It is messy, but so much fun! For a Caribbean beach party we made a collage with handprints turned into big fishes by a few touches of a black pen, and the fingerprints became shoals of tiny fish. We have also used this technique to create individual Christmas cards (see page 74). If you can get hold of a heat embossing gun, ink and powder, use the inky fingerprints to create baubles on a tree shape, or robins on a twig, then add the powder, heat with the gun and create raised glossy decorations!

- One lady, previously an abstract painter, was no longer able to sequence painting, even with extensive support. So instead I gave her a selection of brightly coloured objects and paper that she organised according to an inner sense. I then photographed and displayed the results.

- Create a group collage around a favourite poem – for example, Wordsworth's 'The Daffodils' or Jenny Joseph's 'Warning'.

- Use a black pen to outline things – it makes a real difference.

- Enjoy the abstract!

- Remember that it is the experience of playing with colour and the sensation of changing things that is perhaps the most important part of the activity.

- Remember to put residents' names on their artwork, take lots of photographs and display the art on the wall!

Sensory art session

This session is a slow means of creating abstract art. I have seen it used very successfully to change the mood of residents from agitated or stressed to calm and centred. It might also be used as a more sensory approach to a regular art session. I would use this in a small group, or in a one-on-one session.

Be careful what you call this session – although you will be using paint techniques taught to anthroposophic art therapy students, you cannot call what you do 'art therapy' unless you are qualified.

NB: I would strongly suggest practising these examples before trying them with others!

Ingredients

- Watercolour paper – you could use regular paper, but watercolour paper is very absorbent and allows the paint to flow differently

- Jars of water

- Saucers, palettes or small pots for mixing paints

- Paintbrushes with wide, flat, bristled ends

- Watercolour paints – tubes of colour are best – pick a couple of colours and stick to them. You will need to water the neat paint down before the session.

Method

» Welcome everyone to the room, and set the mood by using music or a poem. Set out the ingredients where you can easily access them.

» Give each person a piece of paper, then bring out the jars of water and the brushes and explain that you are going to practise a particular way of painting. Before you get the paint out, explain that you are going to practise using water. Demonstrate the stroke you want – use a brush full of water and start in a top corner of the paper. In a continuous action move the brush across the paper to the other top corner. This is a slow and concentrated action, not a swift movement – slowness and concentration help to create focus. Work from the top of the paper to the bottom, just using water. This is not only a chance to practise brush strokes, but a very important part of preparing the paper to take the paint.

Palette paint is fine, but if you want to stick to one or two colours, you need to be very clear in your instructions

- Means of protecting work surfaces – plastic table cloths or a board on which to put the wet paper (one per person)

- A quiet room with no distractions

- A CD (and CD player), perhaps of relaxing music, or birdsong; or a poem to set the mood

- Residents who might find this beneficial

» Having previously selected a set of colours (two to four is ideal) get out the first colour (try red). Using the same action, apply the paint to the paper. From here you can branch out in as many directions as there are paintings, but for a first time, work from the top of the page down to about two thirds. Remove the first colour and give out the second colour (try blue), using it in the same way, working up from the bottom to just below where you ended with the first colour. Finally, using a third colour (try yellow) paint one or two stripes across the gap in the centre of the page, allowing the yellow to blend itself into both the blue below and the red above. NB: The more water you add to the paint, the paler the colour will appear on the paper. Use paler colours for this example.

» Next, try using stronger colours. Using stronger versions of the same three colours, start with yellow in the centre of the page, then blue above and below, and finally the red overlapping the blue and yellow.

For both the paler and stronger colour examples there was no source material, just the act of placing the paint on the paper. The piece pictured in Figure II.1 was created in a group when residents were shown some sunrise and sunset pictures as a starting point. I put the pictures away before we started to paint, as we were not trying to copy things. We used red, blue and brown, and as well as using the basic brush stroke, one resident chose to place spots of colour that spread to become scenery. (The white marks at the sides are where tape was used to hold the paper to the table to meet this resident's needs.)

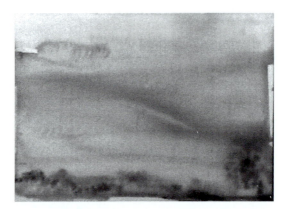

Figure II.1 Veil painting landscape

If you are interested in this style of painting, type 'veil painting' into an image search engine and enjoy the results – or check out some of the galleries listed on page 192. If you type 'art therapy' into the same search engine you will discover all sorts of art styles – art therapy may be the art-making process as therapeutic in and of itself or using psychoanalysis and art as a way to deal with hidden issues.

A group colour layered painting

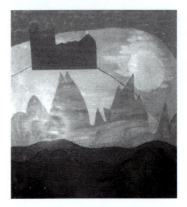

Figure II.2 Group layer painting

This session was used to promote a group feeling of working together, and to work with people who did not consider themselves 'artistic'. The painting required is very straightforward, but the discussion and exploration can involve everyone. The end result is a picture made up of shapes cut from different pieces of paper and 'layered' together on a backing sheet.

Ingredients

- Large sheets of paper
- Poster or acrylic paints
- Large paintbrushes
- Jars of water
- Scissors and a marker pen
- Source pictures
- Saucers or containers to hold paint

Method

» Look at a selection of source pictures – I picked landscapes of various types as appropriate to the group, aiming for simple shapes. We talked about what made up each picture, what appealed to us, and what we disliked, and then discussed our favourite colours.

» As people select their favourite colour, give them a piece of paper and the appropriate colour and paintbrush. Ask them to paint the entire sheet of paper in their chosen colour.

» Lay the sheets on a table, layered one on top of the other, as you plan to cut them to the picture. When you come to mark up the sheets for cutting, make sure that there is a lot of under lap so that layers can be stuck to each other. Mark up the sheets as layers of the picture you have selected. Echo the basic shapes; don't get bogged down in the details. If you are not sure what to keep in and what to leave out, hold the picture at a distance and see what leaps out at you.

» Ask residents to cut along your marked lines if they are able, then layer the sheets one above the other again, and stick them together using sticky tape on the back. If you can, find a frame in which to display the artwork – framing can make all the difference. If not, you could use some black paper to make a border.

Heat-embossed Christmas cards

Helping people to create slick-looking pieces of art is always a challenge, but this technique can create a really professional finish for people working on a very sensory level. I work one-on-one with this technique. You can use this with a high-level group, but you will need to think about sharing a heat gun and embossing powders around the group. Supplies are available from most craft shops these days or you can order them online. NB: If you are working over a bed, use an extra sheet to protect the bedclothes from the embossing powder.

Ingredients

- Card blanks – regular squares or rectangles, or die-cut shapes, e.g. Christmas trees
- An ink block (the colour does not matter)
- Embossing powder in a variety of colours
- Newspaper
- Heat embossing gun – a hairdryer will work at a push, but do not use a DIY heat gun as it is far too hot!

Method for Christmas tree card

» Use a pre-cut Christmas tree shape card. Dip fingers in the ink and make finger marks on the tree shape.

» Working over newspaper, sprinkle the tree with embossing powder so that it covers all the ink marks. Shake the excess powder onto newspaper and return to the pot.

» Use the embossing gun to gradually heat the powder. You will be able to see the powder gently melt and become a slick embossed piece of paintwork – it is fascinating to watch!

Method for robins in the snow

» Dip fingers in the ink and paint a few prints on the card.

» Work with red embossing powder and the method described above; emboss the robins.

» Dip fingers in white paint and paint freely on the rest of the card to create the snow.

» Use a black pen to add the highlights and definition.

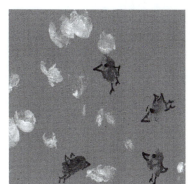

Figure II.3 Embossed robin Christmas card

Making a friendship quilt

This session can help people with different abilities to work to create something together. It can also be used during one-on-one time. Working with fabrics rather than paper and paint brings very different sensory experiences to the group – and can be a real tonic to many women who have knitted and sewed for much of their lives.

Ingredients

- Brightly coloured felt material in lots of different colours

- Ribbons

- Buttons

- Scraps of fabric

- Glue and scissors sharp enough to cut fabric

- Felt-tip pens

- Cardboard templates, about 6 square inches

Method

» Unpack the fabric across the table – and give everyone the chance to enjoy the colours and textures. Use this opportunity to talk about the fabric, and any sewing or craft projects they bring to mind.

» Ask people to select a favourite colour from the pieces of felt.

» Ask them to draw around the templates with the felt-tip pens (use a colour that will show up well). Encourage everyone to line the templates up to edges and corners – this way you will get more from your fabric. If some people need extra support – a hand to hold the template steady, or someone to do the actual drawing for them

- Hole punch
- Needles and thread

— see if another resident can help them out, getting everyone to work as a team.

□ once drawn, the squares will need to be cut out. Felt is good for this, as it should cut easily without sliding around too much. However, make sure your scissors are up to the job before you start.

» Use the hole punch to make a hole in each corner of the squares, but not too close to the edge. These will be used to join the finished squares to one another.

» Encourage people to decorate the squares depending on their preferences and ability. Sorting brightly coloured buttons and sticking them in place, embroidering their name, cutting shapes from fabric scraps and gluing or stitching in place will all look good. This is the time when more one-on-one work can happen – take squares to people's bedrooms and get them involved; suggest themes, objects or events from a person's life story that could be represented. If people are able and would enjoy it, suggest that they blanket stitch around the edge of their square. Encourage people to help one another.

» When the squares are completed, pick pieces of ribbon to tie the corners of the squares together. Lay the pieces flat on a table to tie them together, or you may tie them too tightly, and they will not lie flat. When cutting the ribbon, cut at an angle – this should stop it fraying.

» Display the quilt on a noticeboard where everyone can enjoy it. If you need to take it apart at a later date, return the squares to

» their makers with a piece of ribbon in one corner so they can be hung up – naming the backs of the squares as they are made will help with this!

» Fabric squares made in this manner can also be used as lavender bags – glue two pieces back to back with dried lavender between them. Or apply them to the front of cushion covers – use iron-on Bondaweb (following the manufacturer's instructions).

Books

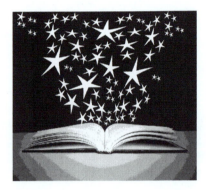

Suggested resources

Selection of books aimed at
adults and children containing
short stories, poetry and prose

Magazines and newspapers

Risk

- Being beaten over the head with a book when you read
  something that interests no one!

Some suggestions

- Either get people talking about rhymes and poems they
  remember and then pick up the book, or vice versa.

- For most people work with familiar things rather than trying
  to introduce new things. Be aware of the different journeys of
  different residents.

- Read a familiar poem aloud and people will often join in – try the 'Owl and the Pussycat', or 'Daffodils' – these are great favourites of ours. Don't be afraid to use props to make your story or poem even more accessible.

- Use the books as talking points, and don't be offended if your Oscar-winning performance is ignored by those around you!

- Encourage those who still can to read aloud – but make sure that the words are large enough and the light is good, and don't forget glasses for those who need them. Don't set people up to fail – if someone starts well and begins to struggle, help them out, or suggest that maybe the print is too small, or the light too poor – give people get-out clauses!

- A group with early dementia found doing play readings of Potted Panto or short Shakespeare plays very enjoyable. We even performed one at Christmas – and hijacked relatives to fill in the parts. We used hats and suggestions of costume rather like Tommy Cooper!

- Allow people to sit 'reading' even if you feel they are not really able.

- Sit and read to someone who finds the sound of your voice comforting.

Cooking

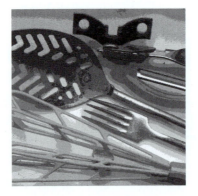

Suggested resources

Flat baking trays

Bun trays

Rolling pins

Mixing bowls

Measuring spoons

Spatulas

Measuring jug

Cake tins

Balloon whisk

Silicone cake/bun moulds

Set of scales

Recipe books

Paper cases

Blunt fruit knives

Pastry brush

Vegetable peeler

Wooden spoon

Plastic spoon

Sieve

Set of shaped biscuit cutters

Set of round biscuit cutters

Greaseproof paper

Ingredients

Risks

- Cross-infection is the biggest risk – remember your food hygiene. Help clients to wash hands before cooking, and don't forget to wash your own! If this is a struggle, try squirting washing-up liquid onto people's hands – rub it in like hand cream, which then feels sticky, and makes rinsing it off fun. Alternatively, use personal care gloves. Make sure you clean the area in which you are going to work.

- If a client has an infection, give them a part of the whole, for example a lump of biscuit mix, and get them to work on just that segment – this can either be disposed of or cooked separately and given to just that client to eat.

- Be aware of sharp (e.g. vegetable peeler) or heavy (e.g. rolling pin) implements.

- Try to keep working areas as clear as possible.

- Remember to store ingredients correctly in airtight containers, or in the fridge.

- Make sure that recipes are checked with the chef first! NB: Do not use raw eggs unless the end product is to be cooked thoroughly.

Some suggestions

- If you are able to take residents to the kitchen, great; if not, bring what is needed to where they are.

- Involve other staff if possible – this helps to avoid accidents. You could also involve relatives.

- Be aware of dietary requirements, for example allergy to nuts, dairy or gluten products, and medication-controlled diabetics.

- Get people involved in steps of the process – one person could measure the flour; another could cream the eggs and sugar. This way you work with one resident at a time, giving them your full attention.

- Don't feel that the end product has to be edible – the sensations of feeling the raw ingredients such as biscuit dough can be just as important!

- If it is safe to do so, allow residents to try ingredients such as fruit or chocolate. When we make something as a group, I have lots of teaspoons with me so that everyone can have a 'tasty lick' of the finished mix before it's cooked.

- If you are particularly interested in the sensory aspect for a resident, consider making up biscuit dough in advance. You can then spend time exploring, manipulating or eating it, as well as rolling it out and cutting out biscuits. Don't forget to smell everything, from cinnamon to treacle.

- In one Home we were not allowed to take residents into the main kitchens, so I either asked the chef to cook something, or had to be prepared to be in the kitchen myself. It's always worth checking that there will be space in the oven, and time for the chef to keep an eye on the cooking. Bribery helps – let the chef try some!

- Alternatively, aim to do 'no cook' cooking, with things that need time in the fridge, or that can be eaten straight away. If you have access to a microwave it may be worth investing in some silicone bowls and cupcake cases.

- Involve residents in 'helping' get lunch – you could ask the kitchen to provide potatoes or carrots that need to be peeled.

- Pick unusual but easy recipes to cook ready for a themed event.

- Why not invite everyone to afternoon tea? Allow different residents to be hosts or hostesses, and try to pick somewhere different to run it – maybe take it in turns to get residents to host in their own bedrooms. Use it as a charity fundraiser and invite other staff and relatives as well.

- Reminisce using cooking equipment – which day was baking day? Talk about people's favourite food – this is also a useful diet tool! Often residents had a 'thing' they were really good at – pastry or cakes, or maybe their Irish stew! What do they remember their mum making? Did they measure ingredients, or go by instinct? Did they ever win prizes at the village fête?

- Don't forget to leave time to wash up – this is an activity too! Check that kitchen tools are safe and clean before storing them.
- Remember that homemade biscuits, iced or not, or sweets make great Christmas gifts when packed in cellophane bags!

For the recipes that follow, refer to the charts for conversions to American weights, etc.

American cup conversions	Imperial	Metric
1 cup flour	5 oz	150 g
1 cup caster/granulated sugar	8 oz	225 g
1 cup brown sugar	6 oz	175 g
1 cup butter/margarine/lard	8 oz	225 g
1 cup sultanas/raisins	7 oz	200 g
1 cup currants	5 oz	150 g
1 cup ground almonds	4 oz	110 g
1 cup golden syrup	12 oz	350 g
1 cup uncooked rice	7 oz	200 g
1 cup grated cheese	4 oz	110 g
1 stick butter	4 oz	110 g
Liquid conversions		
1 tbsp	½ fl oz	15 ml
⅛ cup	1 fl oz	30 ml
¼ cup	2 fl oz	60 ml
½ cup	4 fl oz	120 ml
1 cup	8 fl oz	240 ml
1 pint	16 fl oz	480 ml

Oven temperatures

Gas	°F	°C
1	275°F	140°C
2	300°F	150°C
3	325°F	170°C
4	350°F	180°C

Oven temperatures *cont.*

Gas	°F	°C
5	375°F	190°C
6	400°F	200°C
7	425°F	220°C
8	450°F	230°C
9	475°F	240°C

Weights

Imperial	Metric
½ oz	10 g
¾ oz	20 g
1 oz	25 g
1½ oz	40 g
2 oz	50 g
2½ oz	60 g
3 oz	75 g
4 oz	110 g
4½ oz	125 g
5 oz	150 g
6 oz	175 g
7 oz	200 g
8 oz	225 g
9 oz	250 g
10 oz	275 g
12 oz	350 g
1 lb	450 g
1 lb 8 oz	700 g
2 lb	900 g
3 lb	1.35 kg

Volume

Imperial	Metric
1 tbsp	15 ml
2 fl oz	55 ml
3 fl oz	75 ml
5 fl oz	150 ml
10 fl oz	275 ml
1 pint (20 fl oz)	570 ml
1¼ pints	725 ml
1¾ pints	1 litre
2 pints	1.2 l
2½ pints	1.5 l
4 pints	2.25 l

NB: A pint isn't always a pint: in British, Australian and often Canadian recipes you'll see an imperial pint listed as 20 fluid ounces (fl oz). American and some Canadian recipes use the American pint measurement, which is 16 fluid ounces!

Some no-cook suggestions
Salad

» Fruit will need prepping, mixing and slathering in cream.

» Green salad will need prepping and mixing.

» Potato salad will need precooked potato chunks to mix with mayonnaise; try adding chopped herbs or spring onions as well.

Use pre-shredded cabbage and carrots to make coleslaw by mixing with mayonnaise; try adding some sunflower seeds or a little onion for an extra twist.

Cucumber sandwiches
Or any other kind of sandwich, but cucumber sandwiches are posh afternoon tea material! Lay thinly sliced cucumber between buttered slices of thin cut bread, and remember to cut the crusts off!

Peppermint creams

Ingredients

- 9 oz icing sugar
- A few drops of green food colouring
- Half an egg white from packet mix (2½ tsp) or use similar amount of water
- 1 tsp peppermint flavouring
- 2 tsp lemon juice

Method

» Sieve the icing sugar to remove any lumps.

» Mix egg white, flavouring and colouring in a bowl, then stir in to icing sugar.

» Mix until dough is formed using your hands.

» On a surface covered with icing sugar, roll out using a sugared rolling pin to the thickness of your little finger, then cut into pretty shapes with small biscuit cutters, or roll into balls and flatten slightly.

» Leave to dry on foil or greaseproof paper for an hour or so.

NB: These can be kept for up to three weeks.

Almond hearts

Ingredients

- 2 oz icing sugar
- 2 oz caster sugar
- A few drops of red food colouring
- 4 oz condensed milk
- 4 oz ground almonds

Method

» Sieve the icing sugar, add the caster sugar and ground almonds, and stir.

» Mix in the condensed milk and food colouring.

» Roll out as for peppermint creams above.

Chocolate fridge cake

Ingredients

- 2 oz butter
- 2 tbsp golden syrup
- 4 oz plain chocolate
- 2 oz raisins
- 1 oz cherries
- 6 oz digestives or other biscuit
- Topping: 4 oz plain chocolate and 1 oz butter

Method

» Put the digestives (or other biscuits) in a plastic bag and tie the handles together. Hit the biscuits with a rolling pin until crushed! Some lumps are fine as they add to the texture, but make sure that there is nothing too big.

» Chop the cherries into halves or quarters.

» Break the plain chocolate into smaller chunks and put into a microwaveable bowl with the butter and golden syrup (consider buying the syrup in a squeezy bottle – much less sticky!) and melt – this takes about 1 minute.

» Mix the crushed biscuits and the raisins and cherries into the melted chocolate mix, then put into a tin about an inch deep, lined with greaseproof paper.

» Break the chocolate for the topping into a microwaveable bowl with the butter and melt. Pour over the cake and put in the fridge for a couple of hours.

» Remove, cut into squares and serve!

» For an alcoholic variety, soak the raisins and cherries in alcohol (such as brandy) before using.

» Try adding mixed peel or marshmallows for a different taste.

Lemonade

Ingredients

- Bag of lemons
- Fizzy water
- Sugar
- Lemon juicer
- Jug

Method

» Halve the lemons and squeeze the juice into a jug.

» Add one tablespoon of sugar per lemon, and top up with fizzy water. Taste before serving.

» For an exotic twist, tear up fresh mint leaves and add to the mix – don't worry if people eat them, but bear in mind the choking risk.

Chocolate cornflake cakes

These can be made using different breakfast cereals such as cornflakes, rice crispies, Weetabix or muesli, but quantities will vary. Try with milk or plain chocolate depending on how sweet the cereal is. Although this is 'no-cook', you will need a microwave to melt the chocolate.

Ingredients

- 2 oz butter
- 4 oz chocolate
- 4 tbsp golden syrup
- 3 oz cornflakes or other cereal

Method

» Melt the butter, chocolate and syrup together.

» Mix the cereal into the melted mix.

» Either spoon the mix into cake cases, or put spoonfuls onto a sheet of greaseproof paper, and leave to set in the fridge.

For a luxurious twist, why not add a little stem ginger with a dash of the ginger syrup in which it is bottled?

No-churn ice cream

This recipe needs to freeze for about six hours – or overnight as a full batch. Smaller bowls take less time. It may need to defrost a little before serving.

Ingredients

- 9 oz icing sugar
- 150 ml whipping cream
- Your choice of flavourings

Method

» Whip the cream and icing sugar together until it forms soft peaks.

» Add the flavouring of your choice, and freeze!

Yup, that really is it! I make a big batch of the base mix, then invite people to choose their favourite flavour and make an individual bowlful which can be frozen with the person's name on it. Add fruit, yoghurt, chocolate, maple syrup – once the flavour is added, whisk it again to make sure it is still holding peaks.

Cooking recipes

If you are able to use a cooker, try the all-in-one sponge cake recipe with variations, shortbread biscuits or scones. The biscuits and scones both work as one-on-one activities, and can even be made in a resident's bed. The cake probably needs teamwork, and could be made to celebrate someone's birthday, or made in fairy cake cases and individually iced.

All-in-one sponge

Ingredients

- 6 oz self-raising flour
- 4 oz butter or margarine
- 4 oz caster sugar
- 2 eggs
- ½ tsp vanilla essence
- ½ tsp baking powder
- Dash of milk
- Buttercream icing: 2 oz butter or margarine, 4 oz icing sugar, jam (traditionally strawberry or plum)

Method

» Preheat oven to 180°C. Grease two sandwich cake tins and line the bottoms with greaseproof paper.

» Traditional method: cream the butter and sugar together, add the eggs and mix well. Add the dry ingredients and vanilla essence.

» Quick method: put everything in a bowl and mix well – this method is easier with an electric beater.

» Add a little milk until the mixture is dropping consistency – i.e. it will drop gently off a raised spoon, but not pour! Split the mix between the cake tins, or spoon into bun cases. Cook for 25–30 minutes, until a knife inserted comes out clean. Turn out of the tins and allow to cool on a wire rack.

» To ice, mix the butter and icing sugar and top one of the two cakes with jam and then icing. Place the second cake on top to make a sandwich, and dust the top with icing sugar.

Coffee cake

»   Rather than milk add 1 dessertspoon of instant coffee dissolved in 1–2 dessertspoons of water. To make coffee icing, use the same quantities of coffee/water, mix in icing sugar until stiff, and mix in a knob of butter. Use to ice the first cake and sandwich the second cake on top, put more mix on top and decorate with halved glace cherries and angelica or walnuts.

Lemon cake

»   Rather than milk add the juice and grated rind of one lemon (or a good slug of lemon juice from a bottle). To ice, use the juice of one lemon and enough caster sugar to make a stiffish mix – this icing sets when poured onto warm cakes or buns. Alternatively, mix up a cream icing as for the coffee cake, using lemon juice rather than coffee.

Chocolate cake

»   Replace one heaped tablespoon of the flour with cocoa powder. Make chocolate icing using melted chocolate, butter and sugar as for the coffee recipe, or make with drinking chocolate.

Shrewsbury biscuits

Although the traditional version of this recipe calls for currants, I use it as an excuse to add spices of various kinds, or perhaps some mixed peel.

Ingredients

- 8 oz plain flour
- 4 oz butter
- 4 oz caster sugar
- 1 oz currants

Method

»   Preheat the oven to 180°C, and line baking trays with greaseproof paper.

»   Cream the butter and sugar, then add the other ingredients and mix well. Leave to chill in the fridge for 30 minutes if possible.

- 1 egg
- Pinch of bicarbonate of soda
- Rind and juice of ½ lemon

» Roll out the dough on a floured work surface using a floured rolling pin to about ½ cm thick. Cut into rounds with a biscuit cutter. Place on baking trays and cook for 20 minutes until golden brown. Cool on a wire rack.

» When adding spices enjoy the different smells; pick one that appeals to everyone, and add a heaped teaspoon. I often use cinnamon, nutmeg, ginger, ground clove or mixed spice.

Shortbread

Ingredients

- 6 oz plain flour
- 4 oz butter
- 2 oz sugar

Method

» Preheat the oven to 200°C and line a baking tray with greaseproof paper.

» Put all the ingredients into one bowl and rub together between the finger tips until everything is mixed in and the mix is the consistency of breadcrumbs. Try not to use the whole hand as the mix will become too warm and the butter will start to get too sticky!

» Form the mix into one ball (called 'pulling together'). Place on a floured work surface and roll out using a floured rolling pin, until about the depth of your little finger.

» Using a variety of different-shaped cutters, cut out the mix and lift the biscuits onto a baking tray.

» Bake for 15–20 minutes until golden brown. Allow to cool on a wire rack.

Macaroons

Ingredients

For each egg white that you use you will also need:

- 2 oz ground almonds

- 3½ oz caster sugar

- ½ tsp almond essence

- Edible wafer paper

- Split almonds to decorate

- Egg white to glaze (you may be able to get cartons of egg white at a local supermarket)

Method

» Preheat the oven to 180°C and place sheets of edible wafer paper onto baking trays.

» Crack the egg gently on the side of a bowl, split the shell and allow the white to dribble out, leaving the yolk behind undamaged. Discard the yolk. If the yolk splits and contaminates the white it will not whisk. Always break each egg separately to minimise risk!

» Whisk the egg whites with an electric whisk (it takes a lot longer by hand), until you have soft peaks.

» Fold the dry ingredients in gently – beating will break down the lovely light froth you've created.

» Put spoonfuls of the mix onto a prepared baking tray, leaving some room for spreading.

» Brush with neat egg white before topping with a split almond (neither of these is essential, but they do look nicer).

» Bake for 20–25 minutes until beginning to colour. Remove from trays and discard (or eat) the excess wafer paper.

» Allow to cool on a wire rack.

Crafts

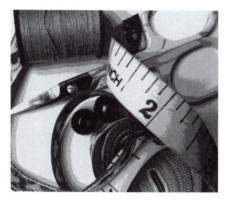

Suggested resources

Glue sticks

Scissors

Sticky tape

PVA glue

Assorted crepe paper

Assorted tissue paper

Glitter

Pipe cleaners

Googly eyes

Card blanks and envelopes

Stickers

Kits, e.g. Easter cards

Ribbon and lace

Beads and buttons

Wool

Paper and card

Felt

Risks

- Scissors and glue are both risky items – use with care, and make sure neither is left unattended. If you have to leave the area, put them away first.

- Small items may pose a choking hazard. Think about who you give them to, and be alert.

- Remember that clients change, and so will their behaviour.

Some suggestions

- Work with only two or three clients at a time, or individually.

- Allow people to explore the textures and colours of the items, and talk about what they see, or how they are used. Pipe cleaners started life as cleaners for pipes – they just turned out to be useful for craftwork!

- Cover tables with a plastic cloth so that it is easy to clean up at the end.

- If you run out of time, keep the half-finished items and plan some more time to finish.

- Don't be afraid to be involved in the making process – think about how you could support a client to complete small parts of the process. Break things down into small steps.

- Play with the buttons – many mums and grandmas had button boxes, which provide a good reminiscence link, and the sorting and sifting can become addictive! Make patterns, photograph them, and then put them back for another day.

- You could make a happiness collage – talk about what makes each person happy, then find pictures in magazines to represent their answers.

- The goggle-eyed monster! For some reason, this is a favourite – the body is made from a small woolly pompom, pipe cleaners are stuck on for legs, octopus style, then googly eyes are added until the individual feels it's complete!

- Make covered notebooks (see page 98), then adapt the pattern to make other things using the same techniques – how about a padded box?

- Use the coloured tissue paper to make cards and displays, or apply it to the outside of glass jars to make pretty candle holders or vases.

- Try *de*construction – this is especially good for those who still have able fingers. I saw this used to brilliant effect at a day centre. Ask families or staff to donate old electrical equipment (but not televisions) – video players are ideal. Use screwdrivers and pliers to take the equipment apart into its component pieces. Sort and categorise them. Use them to make a collage! Be aware of people's abilities and ask for support of a maintenance staff member if available. And cut electric plugs off before you start – you really don't want anyone accidentally plugging anything in!

- Remember that the process is just as important as the end result. Plan an end product, but be open to change if you receive suggestions from the group.

- Remember to put residents' names on their work and take lots of photographs!

Suggestions of things to make

Paper flowers	Table centre pieces
Decorations, e.g. paper chains	Collages to go on the wall
Seasonal, birthday and anniversary cards	Reminiscence work, e.g. a table mat for a client using pictures from magazines, or copies of favourite photographs

Stained glass tissue paper work

This method of working can be used to create all sorts of finished products and artwork on lots of levels. I have used it to create Christmas card designs, window art for theme days, individual pieces around what makes someone happy, or group pieces, specific designs or abstracts. The differing colours of paper make the activity very sensory, and people with little or no artistic ability or fine motor skills can produce stunning results.

One way of working is to use a pattern drawn out on plain paper and slipped under the plastic to use as a template; another way might be to create single sheets of one colour that can be cut up to make a design. Similarly, one person might choose to cut very specific shapes from tissue to make a very structured piece, while others might prefer to rip the paper and create a much more layered and textured piece. Whilst all approaches work, I personally enjoy the ripped and layered look!

Ingredients

- Tissue paper in a variety of colours
- Paintbrushes or glue spreaders
- Source material such as magazines
- Blank paper
- Pens
- PVA glue mixed with water in small pots, e.g. old yoghurt pots
- Clear plastic (A4 polypockets cut open and laid flat, food bags or bin liners)

Method

» Spend time talking to people about what they would like to produce. If there is an end product in mind, talk them through this. Show a part-finished piece so that it is easier to grasp what you are asking people to do. If you are offering source material for people to copy, allow time for them to look through different designs and encourage people to choose something that really appeals to them, rather than something that is 'easy'.

» If you are using a template design (e.g. fish for a seaside theme day), draw this out on plain paper and tape it to the table.

» Tape the clear plastic over the top of the design, or just straight to the table if no design is to be used. If you are using a table that will need to be cleared before you have finished working, use boards or pieces of cardboard to tape the plastic to.

» Mix the PVA glue with water – about half and half, so that it's nice and runny.

» Ask your clients to choose different colours of tissue paper and start them off either ripping or cutting the paper.

» Apply the PVA glue directly to the plastic (it will roll together into beads, and this is fine); then put the tissue paper on top. Brush more PVA glue on top of the tissue. Don't worry about going over the lines of a design – tissue can be trimmed back when it's dry or the lines can be gone over with a black marker pen.

» Work together and don't be afraid to get messy! Use aprons to cover clothes, and have a damp flannel or some paper towels to hand for wiping sticky fingers.

» When you need to stop, or reach the end of a piece, put it aside to allow to dry – timings will vary depending on how much glue you've used and how warm the room is...

» When the piece is finished make sure that people are present when you peel off the backing plastic – this is the magic bit! Hold it up to the light together, or take it to a window and make sure the person can see you.

» Consider making frames out of coloured cardboard for picture pieces, and display on windows with Blu Tack – this peels off the design easily, unlike sticky tape.

» If you are working with several sheets of single colour, cut them up to make a design, overlap the cut edges slightly and use the same gluing method as above to join the sheets.

» If photographing the pieces, remember that the camera will see light differently to you, and allow yourself time to play about with getting it right. Consider using digital images uploaded to an online printing site (such as www.vistaprint.co.uk) to make professional cards.

Covered notebooks

Much of the craftwork we do uses paper, but this is a great project that allows us to get our hands on fabric again. For people who often made their own or their family's clothes, this can be a real pleasure! Although it is a feminine project, with the right type of fabric and magazines, it could easily become masculine as well! There is no sewing involved, so it is not too challenging on specific memories – although if you have people who are good at needlework, knitting or crochet, bring their skills to this project as well.

Ingredients

- Fabrics in a variety of designs (not too thick or stretchy as these are difficult to work with)

- Cardboard

- Scissors that will cut fabric easily

- Marker pens

- Glue (ideally something stronger like an all-purpose adhesive, such as UHU, but PVA will do)

Method

» Create three cardboard templates – one for the finished size you want your notebook to be, one an inch bigger all the way round, and one about half an inch smaller all the way round – templates A, B and C. A good size for template A might be half a sheet of A4 – it will be dictated by the size of the blank paper you have available (e.g. readymade notepads), or by the aims of the project (we made notepads for Operation Christmas Child, so they had to be small enough to go inside shoeboxes...). The smaller the notepad, however, the more fiddly some of the gluing will be.

» Each notebook needs a front and back cover, so this procedure must be repeated twice.

- Plain paper
- Magazines
- Ribbons
- Buttons and other pretty trimmings
- Hole punch

Use template A to cut a cardboard cover. Use template B to cut fabric to go over the cover – place the template on the fabric, draw round it with a marker pen, then cut it out.

» Put PVA or UHU glue all over one side of the cardboard cover, and then stick it to the wrong side of the fabric, getting it as central as possible. Place it so that the fabric is right-side down on the table, and the stuck-on cardboard is on the uppermost side. Put stronger glue if it is available, or PVA if not, onto the fabric that is showing around the cardboard.

» Working on one side at a time, turn the fabric over the cardboard and stick down, overlapping the corners. If you feel confident, trim the corners before gluing (see the figures below).

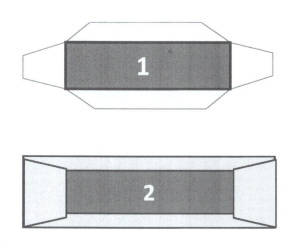

» Use template C to mark up and cut a piece of fabric of a different colour or design to stick over the part of the cardboard that is still visible – it should also overlap with the edges of the first piece of fabric as shown – this is the inside of the cover.

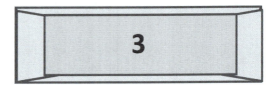

» Leave the cover to dry. If possible, press it flat, otherwise it will curl up during the drying process.

» Use a hole punch to make holes in one of the shorter edges of each cover.

» Decorate the outside of the front cover with buttons, scraps of pretty fabrics or ribbons, crochet motifs or similar.

» Make pages for the book out of blank paper, and hole punch the edges as for the cover. Use magazines to find pictures to stick on some, but not all, of the pages.

» To make up the notebook, place the front cover, outside down, on the table. Place the pages on top, putting plain pages between the decorated ones, and with the front of each page down towards the table, line the holes up. Place the back cover on top of the pile with the outside uppermost and the holes lined up. Thread pretty ribbon from the back cover down through one set of holes of the pile until you have gone through the front cover. Using the other end of the ribbon, work down through the other set of holes in the same manner. Turn the pile over so that the front cover is uppermost. Pull the ribbon tight and tie in a bow.

» Congratulate yourselves on a job well done!

Daily Living

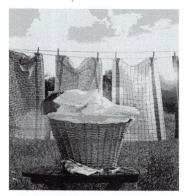

From the moment someone wakes up to the moment they fall asleep at night, the steps that take them through the day can be done *with* them, or done *to* them. The plan here is to try to make every moment a *with* moment. Both Maslow and Kitwood (see pages 23–24) talk about the need for *meaningful occupation*. This section is about the things we have all done every day of our lives. Taking these tasks away from us reduces us to the status of guests in our own home.

Suggested resources

Co-operation and support of people from other departments where you work

Household objects that are familiar to people

Risks

- With the best of intentions, you may end up getting people to do things they don't want to do, or are unhappy doing – but they will soon let you know though!

- Trips and slips when moving around the Home.

- Task-specific problems.

Some suggestions

- When you help someone get up, get them to open the curtains. Talk about the weather – even if neither of you are British! Involve them in making the bed, and talk about all the chores they remember doing as a child to help at home – did they have to earn their pocket money?

- Ask residents to help you lay the table for meals, even if they are only able to lay out their own cutlery from their wheelchair. Don't worry if things don't look 'right' – you can always provide extra things or pass people the right cutlery when the meal starts.

- If possible, encourage residents to help make, or hand round, snacks and drinks.

- Ask the receptionist or administrator to let a resident help deliver papers or the post – use a trolley if necessary, or how about a postman's bag?

- Ask the laundry to save you towels, tea towels, aprons and tabards to fold. This will make their day easier, and may even earn you brownie points! Pairing socks is also fun! If you run out of resources, raid the linen cupboard and unfold the towels, or borrow someone's selection of socks. But be prepared to put things right later if necessary!

- Ask the kitchen for simple vegetables or fruit to prepare – and remember your food hygiene when doing this task.

- Encourage able residents to help with vacuuming, but think through who you ask to do this, as some modern vacuum cleaners are very heavy. Consider buying a carpet sweeper.

- Polish the silver, or the stainless steel. I have an understanding with a local stallholder at a flea market – every couple of weeks she lends me a pile of cutlery, we polish it and then return it for her to sell. Some charity shops are happy to do this as well. NB: Silver is easier than brass to polish – silver polishing cloths are readily available, but brass still needs a good dollop of brass cleaner.

- Dusting is an absorbing activity – one lady I knew would put on an apron every morning after breakfast, with at least one duster in the pocket. She would then happily start to dust the unit, which was circular. When she got back to her starting point she had forgotten where she had begun, and would go round again. We kept an eye out, and if she started to look tired, we would break for elevenses no matter what the hour.

- Washing and drying up are lovely sensory activities if you add lots of bubbles. It's much better to use real crockery and cutlery, even if it needs rewashing again later, but plastic plates can be used, particularly if the resident has weak hands or wrists. You could even take a bowl of soapy water to a resident in bed, or at a table, and ask them to wash up there.

- Wash dolls clothes or personal underwear together – but bear in mind basic hygiene. Install a clothes line or a clothes horse, and peg out the washing to dry.

- Bring in flowers to arrange, or get hold of silk or plastic ones that are not going to mind any rough treatment. Enjoy the smells or different textures.

- Water the pot plants – use pots of herbs as a table centre, which provides a great smell and are edible too! If silk and plastic plants start to suffer, use saucers under the pots, then add water to the saucer and not the plant (oh yes, this one hates to get his leaves wet!). Extra water can be tipped away later.

- Talk about 'women's work' – one lady used to tell me, 'A man's work is from morn to set of sun. A woman, poor creature, her work is never done!', although sometimes we had the rude version! The gents respond well to my comments about how well trained they are, and how I *love* a man who does his own washing up!

- Ask the gardener or maintenance person for help – could they support someone to feed any pets, weed borders, mow the lawn, sort tools, count screws and nails, etc.? Remember that not everyone spent their lives doing housework, so try to think about activities from people's past working lives that might make them feel they have a continued 'worth'. Does the administrator need stamps sticking on or envelopes stuffing – particularly if you are mailing out invitations to an activities event?!

- You can take most of these activities to people who are in bed – chop onions to create a smell for someone, or wash cloths with them, immersing their hands in soapy water.

- Remember that the most important part of these activities is feedback – if someone always hated housework, no longer wants to be busy 'at work' and is pleased to be retired, don't force them to do things. Watching can be an activity too. At the same time, watch out for people who get so involved they don't know how to stop and keep going to the point of exhaustion. And there are also plenty of people who moan incessantly, but who hate not being busy – moaning or grumbling is part of how they do the job, so don't be fooled!

- Allow people to 'help' you – either truly providing assistance, or being part of something to the best of their ability. Either way, praise them for their support – nothing much makes us feel better about ourselves than helping someone out and being genuinely thanked.

Exercise

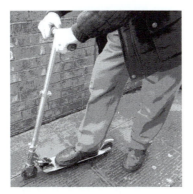

Suggested resources

Balloons

Nintendo Wii

Exercise DVD or instruction set
aimed at this particular client group

Selection of balls of various sizes
and textures, e.g. stress balls, spiky
washing machine balls, soft volleyballs
(a Vitalyz pack is worth investing
in as it will include all of these
as well as other things, designed
with our residents in mind)

Parachute

Dog!

Scarves to wave to music
or to dance with

Whilst all these would be good to have, exercise can be done with
no resources at all.

Risks

- Care Home residents are frail as a group, so care should be taken to make sure they stay safe even while you challenge them – think about balance, flexibility, fragility, vision and diagnosis before you start an exercise group.

- Ideally, go on a training course that teaches you the basics, and certifies you safe to work in this area. Don't be afraid to have a go if you have no training, however – just be careful!

Some suggestions

- Ask people how they feel before you start a session – find out about any new aches and pains, and preference for an upbeat or a relaxing session.

- Always warm up with some gentle breathing and stretching.

- Bat a balloon around – this is surprisingly effective, as even if initially people see it as childish, they can't help joining in! No real force is needed to keep the balloon moving, so it's low impact for fragile joints and muscles, but gets people stretching and moving. This can be used very effectively one-on-one in bedrooms.

- If you are using resources such as balls or scarves, ask residents to help you hand them out and collect them up as this reinforces independence, and also gets people moving.

- Join people who walk a lot anyway, and be part of their usual walk – or get them out into the garden.

- If you are allowed a dog (make sure you check before you ask someone to bring one in, as many companies have rules about animals) take it for a walk. PAT (Pets As Therapy – www.petsastherapy.org) may be able to help with this as their volunteers and animals are vetted and insured.

- Use spiky balls to encourage poor circulation by rolling gently over affected areas. Give someone a really nice shoulder massage by putting the ball behind a resident against the back of the sofa so they can use it themselves, or put the ball on the floor and encourage residents to roll their feet across it – this is great for staff as well!

- Use stress balls to encourage finger flexibility.

- Use larger soft balls to do lift exercises without weights, or place heels or hands on the balls and push backwards and forwards to encourage joint mobility.

- Be brave and exercise the pelvic floor muscles! This is great for improving continence, but difficult to explain. For ladies it's the feeling associated with stopping yourself weeing, for gents the feeling as you walk into cold water and you tense away from it. Get residents to clench and relax, but not too far!

- Want to weight lift? Use individual drinks bottles – either full or empty depending on abilities!

- Join an exercise class yourself, something low impact that gives you transferable skills – Tai Chi or Pilates can both offer something, and that way you'll feel the benefit too.

- Look around for people who offer professional classes in care settings. At one Home we used a gentleman who ran Tai Chi with residents once a month – they wanted him to come much more frequently than we could afford!

- Use the Wii – Vitalyz offers help to set it up for less able residents.

- Put music on in the background – vary between upbeat or sing-a-long and quiet, relaxing music. Something with a beat gives you a structure to do repetitive exercises against, while relaxing music is better for breathing exercises.

- If you feel brave, run a guided meditation session (see page 108).

- Remind people to breathe at intervals during an exercise session – some concentrate so hard they start going blue!

- Some people may benefit from a personal assistant during a group session, either due to comprehension, vision or other problems. Work one-on-one and mirror each other – treat it almost like a dance. If you have clients with a wide range of abilities try running several different classes – gentle, moderate and extreme exercise!

- Why not do a sponsored walk for charity? Get sponsored for the number of metres you can cover as a group, and set up an easy route around the building. Set up a measured metre course in a large room and ask for help to get very frail individuals walking. A sponsored event involves lots of cheering, so everyone feels valued for their contribution! Set up a route around a unit and play upbeat music with a strong beat, get everyone walking in the same direction and go as a group. Allow people to drop out as they get tired.

- Check out the relevant books in the Resources section at the end of this book for exercise programmes, but always try things out on yourself first so you know how it feels and how to lead it. Always start with a few repetitions of an exercise and build up gradually over time.

- Accept the fact that from time to time someone may strain something, or fall when walking. It happens in life, and in the best exercise classes. Just don't let it put you off.

I had wanted to start an exercise programme for a long time, but didn't know how. In the end it came out of a reminiscence session at New Year when my clients and I talked about our resolutions and how we always said we wanted to get fit and lose weight.

Guided meditation

We cannot know what it is like in someone else's head, whether they have dementia or not, but as a person's inner life becomes more real, and the present moment is interpreted through events from a person's past, then it would suggest that visual imagination may remain intact for many people for a long time. This is a different way of connecting to that inner life, one that may well tie in with a person's spirituality.

Meditation is a good way of creating quiet space to 'just be' in a day. Even if some of the people you are working with have receptive aphasia (they are not able to understand the specific words spoken), your tone of voice, manner and body language may provide enough guidance to make this meaningful.

See also the Presence Care Project in the Spiritual and Religious Resources section later (page 200).

Ingredients

- Bravery – it took me a long time to feel confident enough to try this, but it does seem to be worth the effort
- Forethought – think through the journey you are going to take people on, making sure you have thought about how to present it to the group (or individual), and how you are going to bring people back at the end. Also think about where and when – it is no good trying to meditate if the tea trolley is about to arrive... You could also use a CD player with relaxing music or birdsong CDs. Try the scripts on yourself before you use them with a group. Experiment with how slowly you need to go – particularly when counting for breathing

Method

» Explain what you are going to do. Acknowledge that it's not for everyone, and that it may feel weird at first. Encourage people to try it, but if it's not for them, to sit quietly and let others experience it.

» If you want to use a background CD put it on; birdsong is particularly good for garden meditation, but don't be afraid to try without any background noise.

Ask everyone to close their eyes – and close yours (try not to peep, just trust!). Use one of the following scripts as a starting point, or create your own. Use a gentle voice, pitched low so that more people have a chance to hear what you are saying. Speak slowly, and leave time between sentences for people to explore images in their mind's eye.

Script one: The garden

Sit comfortably with your feet on the floor, and your back against the back of the chair. Let your hands rest gently in your lap. Close your eyes and relax. Notice your breathing, in and out. Slow your breathing down so that you can breathe in 2, 3, 4, and out 2, 3, 4. In 2, 3, 4, out 2, 3, 4. As you breathe in feel the air coming into your lungs, then the oxygen heading out around your body. As you breathe out feel the stale air leaving your lungs again. In 2, 3, 4, out 2, 3, 4.

Imagine that you are walking into a garden. It may be a garden that you have been to before, or a new garden that you would like to explore. Take time to look around you. What season is the garden in? Is it fresh and spring-like, with new leaves on the trees, and bulbs emerging, or is it warm summer? Maybe it is autumn, with golden colours and crisp fresh air, or frosty winter.

Look around at what you can see. Notice the colours. The shapes of the plants and trees. The way the sunlight catches different plants. Listen to the sounds around you. Are the birds singing? Can you hear the wind stirring the leaves on the trees? A lawnmower in the distance? Is there a fountain or stream splashing nearby?

What can you smell? A bonfire? Fresh mown grass? The scent of the earth?

Taste the air.

Feel the sun on your face warming you. The breeze lifting your hair. Can you feel the grass beneath your feet?

Take time to explore your garden – follow the paths that wind to hidden spaces, sit on the swing, or just enjoy the peace of the place.

This garden will be here for you whenever you want to come back. Take a last look around now, breathing in how it makes you feel.

We are going to come home now. Let the garden image fade in your mind and concentrate again on your breathing. In 2, 3, 4, out 2, 3, 4. Think about where your body is sitting. Feel the seat beneath you, the floor beneath your feet. Remember the people who are sitting beside you.

As you breathe, wriggle your toes and your fingers a little.

When you are ready, open your eyes and join us in the room.

Script two: Journey to the stars

Sit comfortably with your feet on the floor, and your back against the back of the chair. Let your hands rest gently in your lap. Close your eyes and relax. Notice your breathing, in and out. Slow your breathing down so that you can breathe in 2, 3, 4, and out 2, 3, 4. In 2, 3, 4, out 2, 3, 4. As you breathe in feel the new air coming into your lungs, then the oxygen heading out around your body. As you breathe out feel the tiredness and tension leaving your body. In 2, 3, 4, out 2, 3, 4.

Imagine that you are above this room, looking down into it. You can see yourself sitting relaxed and at peace, with others around you.

As you breathe in you are rising up gently until you are above this building. You can see it set in its grounds, the corridors leading out from where we sit.

As you breathe in again you rise higher until you can see our Home here inside our community. You can see the roads that lead out to other people who live near.

Breathing in you are able to rise higher until you see our town as part of our county, all the different places joined up, linked together, and between, the fields, the open spaces.

As you rise higher again you are able to see our whole country spread below you. Take time to notice that you can see other places that have been special to you. We are not going to visit them now, but you can see that they are all connected together. The whole island looks like a jewel, set in the blue of the ocean.

You rise higher again. Now you can see how our country fits into the rest of the world. Even here you can see the lines made by planes and ships, by letters and telephone calls as they connect all the different parts of our world together.

Now you are going to rise higher again.

Our planet is far off, one of many moving gently in the heavens. You are free here. Held safe in the blackness of space.

Allow the things that have been troubling you to drift away. Know that here you do not have to worry about these things. Here you can be at peace.

Allow yourself to rest.

It is time to go back now. Breathe in the sense of peace and freedom you have found, so that you can take it with you. We are going to journey back together, but there is no hurry.

As you breathe in you move slowly towards our planet. It comes gently towards you.

As you breathe in you are sinking slowly towards earth.

Breathe in and see the countries laid out below you.

As you breathe in you sink gently towards our country, surrounded by the sea.

Breathe in and see the counties become distinct.

As you breathe in you can see our county below you. As you move closer you can see the different towns and villages.

As you sink gently you can see our town.

Moving down you see our Home below you.

As you breathe in you come down through the building until you are above yourself here in the room.

As you breathe in again you are back here. Take a moment to think about where you are sitting. Feel the seat beneath you, the floor beneath your feet. Remember the people who are sitting beside you.

As you breathe, wriggle your toes and your fingers a little.

When you are ready, open your eyes and join us in the room.

Don't worry if people don't want to come back, or doze off – just let them be, they'll re-join you when they're ready.

Head to toe seated guided exercise session
Ingredients

- A group of residents who are keen to give it a go!
- The sheet of instructions for the first few sessions until you feel confident – with thanks to Jo Markham-David who produced a version of this programme that I used for many years (start with some gentle warm-up breathing and stretches; this session looks low impact, but even when I was walking a mile to and from work each day I felt the benefit of running this session!)

Method

Ask everyone to sit up straight, with bottoms far back in the chair and feet flat on the floor. Some people will need a cushion behind them (if they have short legs), or the foot plates of their wheelchair will need to be removed. Use the following instructions.

» Pull in your stomach, and imagine that there is a piece of string attached to the top of your head which is pulling you upwards and straightening your spine.

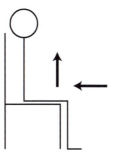

» Shoulder circles: roll your shoulders in big circles starting by lifting them up towards your ears, then rolling them back, down and forwards. Repeat five times.

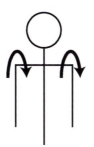

» Shoulder lifts: lift your shoulders slowly to your ears, then drop down – feel free to sigh or groan as you drop them! Repeat five times. Try not to tense your shoulders at the top of the lift, as they may cramp.

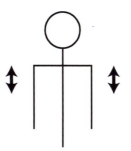

» Arms overhead: lift one arm above your head; try to straighten it without lifting your shoulder! Change arms and repeat. Then if you can, link your hands in front of you and gradually lift them together above your head – again trying not to lift your shoulders! NB: This may be difficult for those who struggle with breathing. Encourage people to stop if it's painful or difficult.

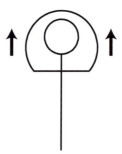

» Back stretch: link your hands in front of you again, but instead of lifting your arms up, push your hands as far away from you as you can, at about chest height. As you lean further forward drop your head between your arms (like a swimmer). Don't overbalance! Gently return to a sitting position, and repeat three times.

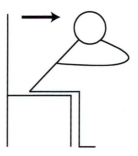

» Chest stretch: sit up tall with your stomach in. Place your hands on your hips, then take your elbows back and squeeze your shoulder blades together – your bust or pectoral muscles will suddenly stick out! Repeat five times.

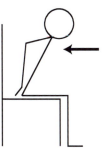

» Chest opener: sitting up straight, bring your arms up to shoulder height in front of you and cross them – as if you were going to dance a hornpipe. Keeping your arms bent and leading with your elbows, slide them sideways until your chest pops out! Slide back. Repeat five times. Beware of hitting your neighbour!

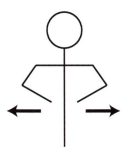

» Shoulder twists: a very gentle exercise that works on the ball and socket joint at the shoulder. Sitting up straight and with arms straight at your sides (or as near as you can get if you have arms on your chair), turn your hands in and out. Repeat five times.

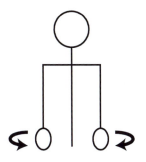

» Elbow twists: bend your arms and tuck your elbows in to your sides with hands palm-side up as if you were carrying a tray. Turn your hands palm-side down, then up. Repeat five times.

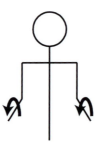

» Wrist circles: trying to keep your elbows still, circle your wrists first one way and then the other. Try for five each way.

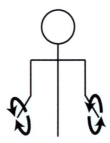

» Sparkly fingers: stretch your fingers so your hands look like star fish, then clench your fists. Repeat five times. Then wiggle your fingers (more like sea anemones this time!).

» Arm swing: sit up tall and swing your arms as if marching, but be aware of what is around you, and try not to bang hands with your neighbour!

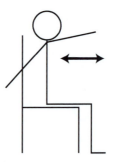

» Trunk rotation: this works best in a chair with arms. Sitting up tall, place both hands on one arm of your chair. Walk your hands towards the back of the chair, turning your body as you go. Walk your hands and turn gently back to centre before repeating on the other side. Take this slowly and gently, going for a maximum stretch that is comfortable. Repeat three times in total, returning to the centre each time.

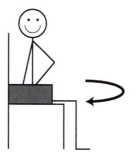

» Buttock squeeze: sitting up tall with your stomach tucked in, squeeze your buttocks together and relax. This gives an entertaining bobbing up and down effect! See if you can find a volunteer to stand in the centre and squeeze their buttocks for entertainment value!

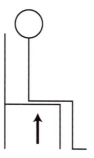

» If you are feeling brave, put the pelvic floor exercise in here from page 107!

» Thigh squeeze: sitting tall with your stomach tucked in, squeeze your knees together and release – this engages the thigh muscles. Repeat five times.

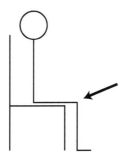

»   Leg stretch: sitting tall with your stomach in, lift one leg off the floor, holding it straight and with your toes pulled back towards your body; hold for five seconds (only lift as far as is comfortable). Put your leg down and repeat on the other side. Repeat again on each side. (When the group is more confident, try holding for longer as well as doing more repeats.)

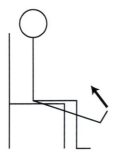

»   Knee lift: sitting tall and with your stomach in, gently lift your knees up and down – as if you are marching on the spot. Go for ten steps (five on each side).

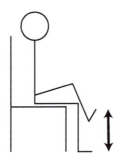

»   Knee circles: great for engaging the ball and socket joint in the hip, but not to be used in the weeks after a hip replacement! Lift one knee in the air and gently draw circles with it. Only do two–three repeats on each side to start with. Repeat on the other leg.

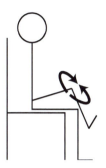

»   Heel lift: sitting tall with your stomach in, lift first one heel, then swap to the other – effectively you are marching but keeping your toes on the floor.

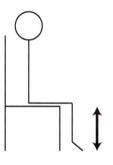

»   Toe lift: the same exercise, but the other part of the foot! March lifting your toes off the floor but keeping your heels down. This is surprisingly hard work!

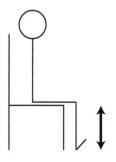

» Ankle circles: using one foot at a time, draw circles in the air with your toes. Repeat five times on each foot.

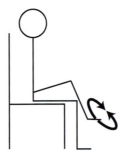

» Ankle stretches: use either one foot at a time, or, if you are feeling brave, both together. Point your toes, stretching the fronts of the ankles, and then bend the feet back towards the body, pulling your toes towards your knees and stretching the backs of your ankles. Repeat five times.

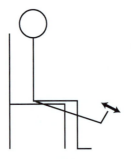

» Neck release: yes you've made it to the feet, now just a few more and we're done! Turn your head gently from side to side – but don't force it! Then gently lower your head sideways so that your ear gets nearer to your shoulder, centre and repeat on the other side. Nod your head gently to your chest. Bring it up again gently.

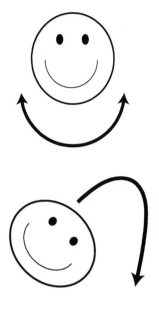

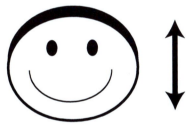

» Spine curls: nod your head gently, and instead of stopping, bend forward so that you curl up into your lap. Rest for a few seconds and then gently uncurl so that you sit up straight.

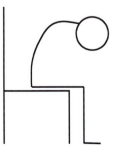

» Finally, roll your shoulders back, give your hands and feet a shake, heave a big sigh (really! this is good for your lungs!) and RELAX!

» WELL DONE! Time for a cup of tea!

Be aware of your group and think about the numbers of repetitions you ask them to do – when starting the session asking for only two repetitions feels like you've hardly explained what to do when you are moving on. By the end of the session those five repeats can feel like running a marathon! Consider using every other exercise in the list so that most bits of the body get a work out, but the overall length is less. As the head to toe approach is repeated week by week the pattern becomes familiar to everyone – if you miss something out someone will soon spot it!

Games

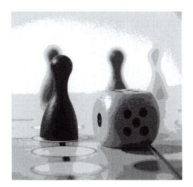

Suggested resources

A selection of games including skittles, dominoes, sorting and matching games, floor games, card games, board games, quizzes, marbles, spillikins (jackstraws), inflatable balls

Small pieces in a box, e.g. dice in several sizes, giant counters, etc.

Risks

- The greatest risk is posed by small pieces, e.g. dice, counters or marbles. These may be dropped and pose a trip hazard, or present a choking risk if swallowed.

- Be aware that some clients may misinterpret things, and use them inappropriately. Be vigilant and offer alternatives, without making the client feel in the wrong.

Some suggestions

- Allow residents to do as much for themselves as possible – give visual prompts to action, e.g. make a shaking and throwing action with your hand as you ask them to throw the dice.

- Add sound effects to games – be prepared to play yourself!

- Don't feel bound by 'rules' – if you can adapt a game, then do it!

- Be happy not to finish something – you don't have to get to the end of a snakes and ladders game for it to have been worth doing!

- Look at parts of the game with new eyes – dominoes can be building blocks; spillikins may be for making patterns or stirring the coffee… Explore the different items as sensory objects.

- Talk about the games if playing them is too hard – chat about childhood and what games individuals remember, whether or not they can explain the rules.

- Be very aware of residents' level of ability, especially when it comes to quizzes. Try 'Tell Me' or something similar: give a category, e.g. girls' names, then a letter of the alphabet. See how many residents can get. Another favourite is to try to get words to do with a theme for every letter of the alphabet. A multiple-choice quiz can also go down well, especially if it is written down, so that people have time to digest what is asked.

- One of the best quizzes is the 'Proverb Game' – start a proverb, pause, and many residents will be able to complete it for you. Test the water by talking about one you can't think of the ending to – ask for everyone's help. Proverbs work well because they are formulaic, and always repeated in the same way, so they stick in the mind. There may be regional differences, however, so stay on your toes. Nursery rhymes can also work well, as do pairs and opposites. Many books have lists of proverbs, sayings and phrases, but have a brainstorm and you'll be surprised how many you find! This can be a good way of involving other staff – run a competition! NB: If nursery rhymes work with your residents, and are enjoyed by them, don't feel you are being childish. Let the residents show what works for them.

- Picture lotto is a better alternative to either bingo or snap – it's a lot less frustrating for the person running the session, and prizes happen more often! It also means there is a lot to talk about if the 'game' process is too complicated.

- Use target games to encourage mobility – throwing beanbags into hoops on the floor, onto a mat or into buckets is good. If some residents find this hard, why not work in teams and go for a team score? Don't forget to spend time choosing a team name... And be prepared to move the targets to and fro to cater for different abilities. Why not go for a 'picnic'? Spend time asking people what they might take on a picnic (I've had suggestions from caviar to loo roll, and everything in between!), then allocate a different item to each target. People can then 'throw a picnic'!

- Be prepared to adapt – we play alley skittles, and I've made an easy-to-remove alley with two bits of wood down the sides. We slant them in so that the ball is always guided to the skittles. We use a piece of guttering to help frailer residents to join in and still get good scores. Skittles sets can be found in all the main supermarkets as summer approaches. Alternatively, put all the skittles in the centre of the room and go round the group seeing how many goes it takes to knock all of the skittles down. Vary the shape in which you set the skittles up. Use several sets of skittles. Put hats on the skittles – get the person who knocks them down to wear the hat (or hats).

- Throw a beach ball around the group – a blow-up one is ideal as it is fairly low impact. Use the throw to each person as an excuse to ask them a question – e.g. what to take on the 'picnic' mentioned above. This way the ball acts as a 'talking stick', giving everyone the chance to be involved in a discussion. You can use the same question for every member of the group, e.g. what would you wear on the beach? Or make every question different. Use knowledge gained in the residents' life stories to prompt questions, or use the exercise to gain life story information!

Themed lotto

We've made several themed lotto games – for Italy, for Nurses Day, looking at emotions, famous faces – the list goes on! Residents had a real sense of achievement that they were playing a game they had made themselves, and we found that if we got bogged down and were unable to recognise the pictures, there was lots of opportunity for reminiscence and discussion around the pictures. The cards we made had nine pictures on each – that way they should fit on an A4 sheet and there are not too many to scan whilst playing, as there is no logic to the layout, unlike a number sequence. If the cards are laminated you can use them with dry wipe markers; if not, plastic milk bottle tops make ideal large playing counters.

Ingredients

- For making: plain paper (preferably a bright colour), glue, scissors, laminated sheets and a laminator, source pictures (approx.18–20 different ones printed out five times each in small prints, plus one of each printed out A4)
- For playing: finished game cards, plastic milk bottle tops (nine per player) or dry wipe marker pens, small prizes

Method for making

» Find your source pictures, making sure they are sufficiently different from one another to show up easily – the internet is the best place to look, although images must be free from copyright. Clipart is another place to look. Save the images to your computer and print them out – most printing wizards allow you to select a 'wallet' setting where it will print out nine images to a page, which will give you the right size pictures. Remember to also print out an A4 version of each picture for you to hold up. Talk to the administrator before you print them out, so that an economical ink setting can be used!

» Ask residents to cut out the pictures.

» Make up the cards by using one blank sheet of paper and sticking on nine different pictures. The aim is to select the pictures randomly so that the sheets all end up different; use each picture only once on any card – 18 pictures printed out five times each will give you enough for ten cards.

» Laminate the sheets so they will last for more than one game. And laminate the A4 versions of each picture.

Method for playing

» Talk about the theme you have chosen for your game. We talked about people's memories of the Coronation when we played Jubilee Bingo!

» Ask everyone to select a playing card.

» Allow time to look at the pictures and talk about them a little.

» Give everyone a dry wipe pen, or nine milk bottle counters.

» 'Eyes down looking for a full house!' Shuffle the A4 cards, and hold one up – if necessary, talk about or describe what it shows. Encourage people to look at their cards and cross off or cover up the matching image.

» Continue until someone has a 'full house'. Encourage them to shout out – you might make up a new call dependent on your theme. We had to shout 'nursey, nursey' for our Nurses Day lotto.

» Check the pictures, and offer a prize.

» Encourage everyone to clean their cards, swapping them if they want. Play again!

Some themes have worked more successfully than others, and it can be hard to tell until you've tried playing to see how it will go. Some of the success lies in what images you choose. If you are able to link with another Home this is a resource you can post easily for them to try out!

Themed beetle drive

This is another game suitable for a themed event, but played as a team. It requires only single steps, so it is good for groups that are less able.

Ingredients

- For making: source pictures printed out A4 size (you will need one per team, with perhaps a few extras to allow for swapping round), plain paper, scissors, marker pen or felt-tip pen, laminated sheets and laminator
- For playing: finished game cards, dice per team, prizes

Method for making

» Using plain A4 paper, draw divisions with a marker pen or felt-tip pen so that the page is divided into six segments, as weird and wiggly shaped as you like. Label each segment from one to six.

» Trim and mount a source picture on the other side of the paper, and laminate together.

» Cut along the marker lines so that each laminated sheet is in six pieces, with each one numbered.

Method for playing

» Give each team a set of six pieces that go to make up one picture, and a dice.

» Encourage the team to take turns to shake the dice and throw a number. As the number is thrown, the piece with the corresponding number is picked up and turned over. For example, a player might roll a 3, so the piece labelled 3 is picked up and turned picture-side up.

» This continues until all the pieces have been turned over – it may take some time! When all the pieces are picture-side up, the team then have to assemble their picture. The first team to do this wins!

» For most themed events each team will then share what they can see in their picture, or read out information from their card.

» To play again, swap the sets between the teams so that everyone gets a chance to make a different picture. Swap spare pictures in and out.

» To make a more complicated version, cut the pictures into 12 pieces, using each number from one to six twice.

» Make up teams that include abler and less able residents, and encourage team working to help break down any barriers.

Gardening

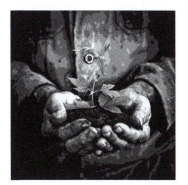

Suggested resources

Earth	Pots
Seed trays	Packets of seeds or bulbs
Seed catalogues, gardening magazines, books about flowers, trees, birds	Garden tools, e.g. trowel, fork, secateurs, broom, twine
(If you are lucky in your grounds, an area set aside for residents, perhaps with raised beds, herb patches, seats, trees, bird table or feeders, window boxes)	

Risks

- Tools are obviously dangerous, and any gardener should use them carefully, but if an individual is unable to remember their proper purpose, tools may be used inappropriately, becoming higher-risk items.

- Be aware of people's journeys and life stories when working in a garden.

- Be aware of other hazards, e.g. slippery paths or the outside temperature.

- There is also a risk that nothing will grow due to over-enthusiastic tending…

Some suggestions

- Start small – you don't need to go into food production and supply the Home with all its vegetables overnight! Be guided by how residents might like to use an outside area.

- Take people out for sensory walks listening to the wind in the trees and the sound of the birds. Bring back leaves, feathers or fruit to share. NB: Make sure you have identified anything that might be eaten – we had deadly nightshade with its shiny black berries in our garden one year.

- Make the outside areas more sensory. Plants with strong smells or colours and edible plants are great, and adding new sounds can also help.

- Just sit and enjoy the garden.

- Chat about what comes next – this works fine in an armchair in the lounge too! Talk about what vegetable you'd like to plant, how rhubarb tends to take over, allotment etiquette, or what flowers would be nice. Use magazines and seed catalogues as props. Allow people to just enjoy the pictures without needing to vocalise. If my mother moves into a Care Home, she will be quite happy to sit poring over seed catalogues for hours, with no need to talk to anyone!

- Remember how important the sensory element of gardening is – sieve soil or mix in additives with the hands (although remember to wash hands before eating).

- Use easy seeds (e.g. cress or 14-day salad greens) to grow things in people's rooms – a tray on the window sill is often better than a window box as most windows have fixed catches. Encourage people to eat what they've grown.

- Plant vegetables in tubs on the patio – I've grown everything from potatoes to runner beans this way.

- Buy magazines with free seeds on the front – or keep an eye on offers in the newspapers.

- Do flower arranging, or try a sensory flower petal massage (see page 158).

- Younger people with dementia are often very physically able, so if it's appropriate, get them to dig and weed in a garden plot, sweep paths or rake leaves. Older people may also be fit and healthy.

- Risk-assess occupations, but try to give people the freedom to pursue their past pleasures.

- Enjoy all the seasons, both outside and inside. Bring in autumn leaves or spring flowers – remember. Do they remember the nature table at school?

- Plant bulbs as gifts for family members.

- Use the art resources to draw what can be seen from the windows.

- Use the craft resources to make attractive plant labels from lolly sticks, or wind chimes from old cutlery.

- Position armchairs or beds so that residents can catch a breeze through the window full of the scent of new mown grass.

- Put on a CD of birdsong in the lounge.

- If you are not garden minded, can you get in a volunteer who loves to garden? This may mean that a resident can be supported to spend hours outside.

- Does your Home have a maintenance person or gardener? Would they like some help? Try to get these people on side – then if someone enthusiastically prunes or digs things up, the damage can be dealt with in good humour.

- Consider entering items into the local produce show – you may not win anything, but it will help with community links.

- Remember to put residents' names on their work and take lots of photographs!

'Inside OUT' poetry

I went to a workshop run by the Wye Valley Inside OUT team (www.wyevalleyaonb.org.uk/index.php/projects/latest-projects/inside-out), who are committed to making their beautiful landscape more accessible to those who might struggle to get there otherwise.

This session is based on the workshop run for us, and reflects the work of the charity. Many Homes are not set up for residents to easily wander in and out, or they must be supervised when going outside. This is one way to bring the outside in. It's also another way to give people permission to be creative – although I don't tend to warn people we are 'writing a poem' the first time!

Ingredients

- Access to the outside world

or

A collection of bits and pieces brought in from the garden – twigs, leaves, grass, flowers, egg shells, moss, feathers, etc.

- Post-it notes

- Pens

Method

» If at all possible, take a small group of people outside. Spend time (well wrapped up if necessary) listening, looking, smelling and touching – use your discretion with tasting! Collect bits and pieces that appeal to people, as mentioned above. Bring everyone back inside.

» If it is not possible to go outside, spend some time collecting bits and pieces before the session. Put a CD of natural sounds on and allow people to explore what you've collected, and choose which items appeal to them.

» Whether you've been able to go outside or not, ask people to look at the things they've chosen, and to arrange them on a piece of paper in a way that is pleasing to them.

- Five sheets of paper, labelled 'Sight', 'Hearing', 'Taste', 'Touch' and 'Smell'

- One large sheet of paper (e.g. flip chart paper)

- Craft materials

Provide craft materials in case people want to use wool or pens and pencils to add to their artwork. Photograph the finished results.

» Give everyone five post-it notes and a pen.

» Supporting people as needed, encourage everyone to write two or three words on the first post-it about what they could see when they were outside; if you were not able to go outside, encourage them to describe times they remember being outside. (You could link this with the garden meditation described on page 109.) Collect the post-its on one of the five sheets of paper labelled 'Sight'. Continue with the other four senses.

» When all the senses have been completed read the words together, or ask a good reader in the group to read them aloud for you. Ask people to string the words together into sentences – start with one sense, and try to use all the words before moving on to the next sense. This might take one or more sentences, and as many extra words or descriptions can be added as needed.

» Read your poem out! Get different people to read it, putting the expression where they feel it needs to be. See Figure II.4 for an example.

» Write the poem out and display it on a board with the photographs of the artwork.

» Finish the session by returning all the bits you collected to the outside world.

Sight
Sunbeams
Rough bark
Tossed leaves

Taste		Smell
Blackberries	Sunbeams catch the tossed	Bonfire
Frost	leaves.	Cooking
Autumn	The ridges of rough bark.	Chrysanthemums
	Sour blackberries shrivel my	
	tongue.	
	I can taste frost, and autumn	
	days.	
	The breeze touches my face,	
	My fingers explore the damp	
Touch	earth and rough bark.	**Hearing**
Damp earth	Bird song echoes around	Bird song
Rough bark	me, mixed with the voices of	Children playing
Breeze	children playing.	Lawnmower
	Far off a lawnmower rattles.	
	Shaggy chrysanthemums hang	
	their heads, smelling like the	
	Church at Harvest.	
	The bonfire sinks and dies.	
	Dinner is cooking, I must be late	
	home!	

Figure II.4 Example of 'Inside OUT' poetry

Wind chimes from old cutlery

Although this is technically a craft project, the end result is designed to be hung outside, and will hopefully enhance people's enjoyment of the outside space. It could be made during the winter months ready to go out in the spring, or made in the garden and hung straight up. This works particularly well with a gents craft group, although you will need to risk-assess whether your residents are able to use the drill, and ask for maintenance support if necessary. You may need to pre-drill the cutlery.

Ingredients

- Old cutlery – preferably metal spoons
- A drill
- Twine or string
- Curtain ring
- Carrying ring (the rim cut from a catering pack of jam, or several wire coat hangers bent out of shape both work)
- A clapper (the lid of a jam jar would work)
- Scissors

Method

» Make sure the cutlery is clean. Drill holes into the flat part of the handles near the ends. I used old cutlery from a charity shop, and it drilled easily. If the spoons are soft enough try bending them into different shapes.

» Drill two holes in the centre of the jam jar lid.

» Using the garden twine or string (this is now available in bright colours from many garden centres) tie the cutlery to the carrying ring. If you are using wire coat hangers you will need to use several tied together, otherwise the weight of the cutlery will bend it out of shape. Space the cutlery evenly around the ring.

» Cut four or more pieces of string the same length. Tie one end of each to the carrying ring, spacing evenly, and the other to the curtain ring. This makes the loop to hang the chimes from.

» Cut one longer piece of string. Tie one end to the curtain ring and post the other down through one of the holes in the jam jar lid, then up through the other. Tie the string to itself so that the jam jar hangs in the middle of all the spoons.

» Use the string or twine to wrap around the visible bits of the carrying ring.

» Hang up in the garden – if you are planting seeds or seedlings out, you could use the wind chimes as a bird scarer.

Knitting

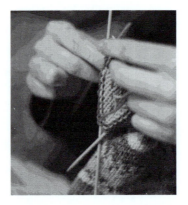

Suggested resources

Pairs of knitting needles

Basic sewing kit – needles
and thread, pins, cotton

Selection of wool, of different
colours and textures (charity
shops often have wool for sale,
or pull apart old garments)

Patterns (for knitting)

Patterns (for reminiscence)

Risks

- Needles may pose a risk as they are pointed. Be selective about
  who you give them to, and where they are put when you are not
  able to supervise.

- Wool may pose a trip hazard. Always be aware of your surroundings, and if you are called away, make sure you leave things safe.

- Pins and needles are small and sharp. Work with them over a tray or table to make sure none are left on the floor or furniture.

Some suggestions

- Get those who can to knit simple strips or squares to be sewn together into blankets (you could link with your local maternity hospital special baby unit or animal shelter to donate finished work). You may wish to keep several needles pre-cast on, as casting on is the most challenging part.

- Use simple patterns with those who can knit, even if you need to tell them line by line what to knit.

- Allow people to do their own thing. One lady knits sleeves – hundreds of them and at some speed too! As her dementia has progressed, the sleeves have got longer and longer, but she always starts with a beautiful cuff! If something ends up a very odd shape, and full of holes, it really doesn't matter – unless it distresses the resident. One very competent knitter actually enjoyed unravelling knitting as her dementia progressed. This was fine as I could spend some time creating long pieces for her to work on, but was a nightmare if she found someone else's knitting left unattended…

- Try winding wool into different balls.

- Help those less able to enjoy the colours and textures of the different wools.

- Reminisce about what things people used to knit, who they used to knit for and who used to knit things for them. Use the reminiscence patterns to talk about different styles or techniques, e.g. Aran, Fair Isle, how to turn a heel, crochet, etc. One lady I know can happily spend hours poring over patterns – she is probably choosing what to make, but never actually reaches that point. She no longer talks, so I can't ask her, but I know it gives her huge pleasure.

- Some people may never knit a stitch, but will still carry a piece around with them (I think it comes under creative displacement activities). I'm about to be very busy with my knitting, but first I've just got time for a cup of tea, or a natter, or a TV programme… Its presence can give a sense of purpose and normality.

- If you can't knit yourself and you have an able resident who can, get them to teach you!

- Don't forget to put residents' names on their work

Knitting patterns

There are some brilliant books on the market to teach you how to knit, from the 'stitch and bitch' books to the 'knitting for dummies' books. The same goes for crochet. You may find that the abilities of those around you vary day to day, or depend on the person not thinking about what they are doing. Knitting is mostly stored with body memories, but the ability to knit particular things has to do with sequencing. Getting someone going on a straight strip is often the best way of starting – and is usually the way we learnt. Who didn't start with a Dr Who scarf? The patterns included below are therefore based on strips and squares, and the relevant books included in the Resources section at the end of this book are to do with making things from these same basic blocks. Why not also try cushion covers, draught excluders or toys? I've also included a description of the four basic stitch patterns just to remind you which is which. To make something smaller, use thinner needles and wool, or cast on fewer stitches and work fewer rows; to make something bigger, use thicker needles and wool, or cast on more stitches.

Basic strip or square

» Cast on 30 stitches. For a strip, knit 18 inches; for a square, knit about 4 inches – until it looks square!

» Cast off.

You could use stocking or garter stitch, or even rib or moss stitch if feeling adventurous!

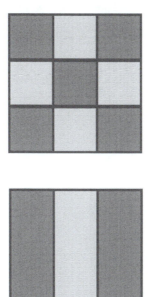

Blankets

» Make three strips and sew them together down the long sides using an over and over stitch.

» Press flat. (This is about the right size for a cot or pram.)

Alternatively, use nine squares sewn in three rows of three.

Egg cosy

» Cast on 20 stitches.

» Use any stitch you like. When the work is seven inches long, cast off.

» Fold in half along the arrow (see below), bringing the short edges together.

» Sew the long edges together with the same colour wool.

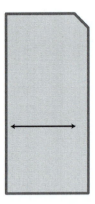

To make the egg cosy, strip or square more decorative, mix colours to make stripes! Knot the old and new colours together before carrying on knitting. Use a large darning needle to sew in stray ends.

Finger puppet

» Cast on ten stitches.

» Work in stocking stitch.

» When the work is eight inches long, cast off.

Fold in half along arrow (see below), match the short edges, and sew the long edges together with the same colour wool. Decorate with buttons or sequins to turn into a person or animal.

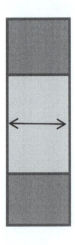

If you are feeling adventurous use two colours – one for the body and one for the head. Cast on in body colour and work three inches, change to head colour and work two inches, and change back to body colour and work three more inches, then cast off. Make up in the same way.

Garter stitch

» Knit every row.

Both sides of the work will be the same, with lines of loops across the work.

Stocking stitch

» Knit one row, purl one row.

Both sides of the work will be different. One side will be lines of loops across the work (usually referred to as the wrong side); the other side will be rows of arrows pointing up and down the work.

Rib

» Using an even number of stitches, for row one, knit one, purl one to end; for row two, knit one, purl one to end.

Rib looks like it sounds – it creates a furrowed effect like a ploughed field – and it is usually used to make cuffs and hems on jumpers. This is 1 x 1 rib – 2 x 2 rib is made using knit two, purl two, and so on. Using more stitches means that each individual furrow is wider.

Seed stitch

» Using an even number of stitches, for row one, knit one, purl one to end; for row two, purl one, knit one to end.

With seed stitch both sides of the work are the same. It can be used for borders and cuffs, and gets its name from the texture of the surface, which looks as if little seeds have been scattered.

Moss stitch

» Using an odd number of stitches, for rows one and four, knit one, purl one to end; for rows two and three, purl one, knit one to end; repeat rows one to four.

This creates a fabric that looks the same on both sides, with a textured effect a bit like the sides of a basket. As with rib, the more stitches, the chunkier the basket effect.

Linking with the Community

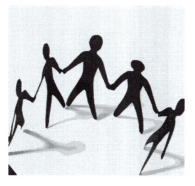

Suggested resources

Phone book

Paper, envelopes and stamps

Charming manner!

Part of what makes us human is our links with other people. It is possible to become very isolated when you arrive in a Care Home. The world can shrink to the few rooms and the relatively small group of people seen every day. As with any other activity, people may need help reaching out beyond their four walls, and this is where linking comes in. There are many different kinds of links – with individuals, including entertainers, with groups locally or further afield, and one- or two-way links. You may have a group that wants to become pen pals with people in another Home, or be kept up to date with world events – ask your group what they want, and try to find something that fits the bill!

Risks

- Potential for miscommunication or being stuck with something that doesn't work.

- Getting more than you bargained for.

- Being let down.

Some suggestions

- Be really clear about what you want to get from a link, or what you want to give. If you aren't certain, be really clear about that. ('We'd like to link with/get to know/work more closely with you, but we're not sure what we can offer, or what you might be able to offer us. Do you have any ideas?')

- Think about your residents and what they would like more of – people dropping in for a chat? Continuing to follow a past interest? Raising money for charity? Seeing people benefit from their wisdom? The presence of children? Music while they eat their lunch? Singing? Working this out will give you an idea of people to contact.

- Make sure you keep copies of any letters or emails so you can check what was promised, and write notes about any telephone calls. Keep everything together!

- Our links tend to be a selection of local schools, each of which has something different to offer; local places of worship and the people who work there; particular entertainers we ask back again; several volunteers – most started as relatives who visited frequently and wanted to give something back after their family member died.

- You will need to go out and find some links – I would really like a choir that can come in and do a sing-a-long, for example; other ideas will be thrown up by residents – 'I used to go to a sailing club just down there, I wonder if we could go and visit?'; and some people will phone up and offer their services. Consider talking to a local Volunteer or Citizens Advice Bureau for ideas on how to meet a particular need.

- Find out your Home's policy about Criminal Records Bureau (CRB) checks for volunteers and insurance policies for visiting therapists.

- Talk to your team and to your manager before you set up a link – especially if it's going to cost money!

Music

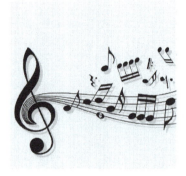

Suggested resources

Song books

Selection of CDs

Selection of percussion instruments – involving shaking, hitting and blowing

Keyboard or guitar complete with someone to play it...

Risks

- There is always a possibility that instruments will break – be aware of the contents of shakers, or sharp edges if this happens, and clear up immediately, binning anything that is broken.

- Clients might react badly to choice of music or the amount of noise. Always be aware of who is in the group, and their reactions. If the main group is enjoying making a noise, try to remove individuals who are struggling to a quiet space, and do something different and quiet with them – don't just isolate them.

- Be sensitive to kinds of music – you may trigger unhappy memories for people.

Some suggestions

- Allow the group to dictate what they would like to do – try to follow up on suggestions, or move away from doing something that is giving a negative reaction.

- Try leading a sing-a-long – and be brave! You don't have to have a great voice, just get the group started and then enjoy being part of it. You could use a CD.

- Be aware that song books might be really good for some people, but not for others – be sensitive to people's levels of reading ability, or ability to find page numbers.

- Use the percussion instruments to allow people to express their own sense of rhythm and enjoyment or to get the group as a whole to experiment with different sounds; get just one type of instrument out at a time or get half the group to use one type, e.g. shaking, and the other half to use hitting instruments – try to get complementary rhythms going.

- Set up a one-two-three, one-two-three waltz time pattern and then sing along with an appropriate song, e.g. 'Cockles and Muscles' or 'How Much is that Doggie in the Window?'

- To experiment with rhythm or singing in rounds, you will need more than one member of staff or a resident who is confident enough to lead one of the voices!

- Music is stored in a different part of the brain to language, so people who can't talk can often still sing. Singing helps the brain to reorganise itself, and may make tasks easier to understand and complete. One lady was unable to remember how to walk, unless we sang 'Onward Christian Soldiers' or something with a similar marching beat – then she was off, singing and marching down the corridor! One lady struggled with personal care, but singing her favourite songs with her whilst this was happening kept her calm and engaged. Sometimes putting simple instructions to music means that the brain can understand what is wanted.

- Many people remember hymns or religious music, as the generation we work with now had a much higher level of church (or similar) attendance. Try and put on music that reaches residents; try downloading hymns recorded by the choir of St Mary's Ross on Wye, for example (see the Resources section at the end of this book). They noticed that although congregations knew the first verse of many hymns, they had no idea about the other verses, yet CDs always include every verse. So on this site they have only recorded one or two verses for each hymn, to keep it user-friendly.

- If you are setting up a concert for a large group, for example carol singers at Christmas, or children from the local school, think about people who are nursed in bed, and be brave about asking groups to move around the Home singing! We ran a corridor concert with a school choir, and reached people who would never have heard it otherwise – and some of the reactions were very deep. The children were also affected – they asked questions about why the people didn't clap and so on, and we ended up having a really interesting talk about what dementia is, and how it affects us.

- We ran a music poll that charted musical interests across our whole Home – residents, staff, relatives, health care, maintenance and visitors – and ran a giant display in reception so that everyone could see what kind of music was in the lead. We asked about previous experience of playing an instrument, what kind of instrument an individual would choose now if there were no barriers, and what sort of concerts people went to as well as favourite types and individual pieces of music. We also welcomed expressions of dislike. Some people couldn't tell us this information, and didn't have friends or family who could help, so in some cases we did quite a lot of research with a CD player! Information was transferred to care plans, and is now used daily, and can really help to inform end-of-life care.

- If using music with someone who is lost very deep within themselves, try getting alongside and listening to their breathing. Start to breathe in time with the person. Use an instrument, for example a rain stick, or use your voice to make a sound every time someone breathes out. Often the person will start to vary their breathing in response. Try it with friends you trust to see what it feels like. As a person responds to your mirroring, try in turn to respond to their changes – if their breathing gets deeper, mirror this by changing the tone or volume of your noise. As you both progress through this journey, start using more than one sound – for instance, hum a phrase for the outbreath. Try to match your sounds to the other person.

- Use this technique with someone who walks a lot. Get in time with their walking, and then use your voice or an instrument to mirror their steps. Pick a song you know and 'la' the tune, one note to every step. Watch for the person changing what they do in response to your mirroring. For more information on either of these techniques contact the Nordoff Robbins Music Therapy Foundation (see the Resources section at the end of this book).

- Consider using a CD player in the bathroom to change a task-led atmosphere to a person-centred one. Make sure that the music on offer is appropriate to the individual.

- As with the 'Proverb Game' discussed above (see page 124), try starting a song title and see if people can finish it. Start the first line of a song – spoken, hummed or sung – and see if people join in. If you know the song, prompt by joining in again whenever anyone gets stuck. See the Resources section at the end of this book for a good music quiz book.

- Be happy to sing just the first verse of things – after all, who actually *wants* to sing all 100+ verses of 'God Save the Queen'?

Reminiscence

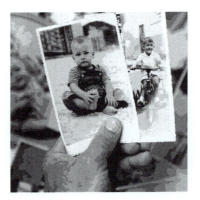

Suggested resources

Photographs or props for any subject from about 1915 to 1980

Family albums and personal property

Risks

- Trying to get someone talking about a subject they have no knowledge of or interest in – usually from the best motives!

- Stirring up distressing memories.

- Asking direct questions for which the resident cannot find a memory or answer.

Some suggestions

- The idea with reminiscence is simply to recall past impressions and emotions. This means that there should be no 'wrong' answer. Don't try to test memories – who is this in the photo? What were they doing? Why? When? Instead, talk about the feelings a picture gives – 'They look happy, don't they?' This might find you information: 'Yes – they were! It's my mum and dad just after they got married.'

- Reminiscence can be a great group conversation starter. We did a big project around the Year of the Child 2009. Every time we met I would bring some pictures of childhood things that got everyone started, and then people would pick up from one another. I only got involved if one or two people started to do all the talking and other people weren't getting a chance – or if the group ran out of words, when I added memories of my own, or started a new topic. People found that they shared lots of memories, and started to form strong friendships based on shared experiences.

- Sensory reminiscence is also possible. I sat with a lady who wept all the time and hardly spoke. I'd thought that Ireland (where she was born) was a good starter, but it turned out that years spent on the Isle of Wight were a stronger memory. I brought a 3D model of the Isle, as well as things like her library card, and we sat together for about half an hour exploring the model with touch and sight, giggling at the photograph on her library card. We did no talking at all, but it was clear that happy and emotional memories were being relived.

- A DVD or CD can prompt memories – try watching old footage of the Queen, or watching a year-specific DVD (the kind you get on birthday cards), and listen to the conversation it sparks.

- Remember that memories are linked to all the senses – smell the spices when you are baking and people will usually start talking about Christmas. The smell of coal tar soap can also be very evocative.

- Consider physical reminiscence using role-play – use Pam Schweitzer's book *Remembering Yesterday, Caring Today: Reminiscence in Dementia Care: A Guide to Good Practice* (published by Jessica Kingsley Publishers in 2008). Pam also suggests drawing reminiscence – start drawing something familiar to the resident and ask for input: 'How many windows?' 'Should it go like this?' I worked with one lady on a picture of how the family kept chickens and how every day the person who used to go round collecting eggs (the heggler) would come and take them to Birmingham market.

- Ask families for old photographs – the earlier in a person's life the better – or ones linked strongly to things they've always enjoyed. Take copies! Losing originals is practically a criminal offence.

- Objects will also bring out strong memories. A lady I know has a broken oar in her room – her husband rowed for his college, and snapped the oar in an important race – it was given to him as a booby prize! The oar's presence brings back this story, which in turn triggers others about her husband. One activities leader told of a resident for whom there was no family, and who wouldn't speak. There was no life story, so everything became a matter of guesswork. Exploring the items in his room, things that were still with him so probably had meanings, the team pieced together his engagement to his one true love who had been killed during a bombing raid in London during the Second World War. The man was prepared to nod or shake his head to suggestions, and when they discovered the right one, he started to talk again.

- Think about how you will store what you learn when reminiscing. If it's topics or prompts that work for a particular person, write them down in the person's notes to jog your memory and so that others can use them.

- Use online tools to create memory books (e.g. www.blurb.com), or if there is no money available, use paper and a glue stick or a downloadable scrapbooking tool. Laminating pages means that books will last longer, and gives it a more professional appearance. You could also consider a comb binder, which your Home may already have.

- With people who are more able, consider using a 'This is Your Life' approach; spend one-on-one time helping them to write the story of their life. Get families involved. Several residents have life story books in their rooms for the family to chat over and to jot notes down in.

- If you are running a group session, make notes on what people say – you can add them to individual life stories afterwards.

- Use a themed reminiscence or rummage kit to lead a session – see 'Rummage' on page 154 for details.

- Reminiscence can be a means to an end – finding out about and creating mementos of a life story – or it can be the purpose – spending time together re-living happy memories.

Rummage

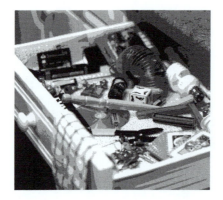

Suggested resources

(These will depend on who the rummage is for, or what the theme is)

Clearly labelled storage containers

Risks

- Providing the wrong thing for a person.
- Items getting put away broken, and causing harm when next used.
- Using heavy or sharp objects.
- Regularly check collections for additions, dirt or damage.

Some suggestions

- Rummage boxes or bags can be provided for a variety of reasons and should contain a variety of things.

- A good general rummage box should contain a variety of shapes, sizes, textures and colours, some items that are familiar, and some that are strange, the idea being that there is a lot to draw you in and keep you exploring. These can be set up and left for residents to dip into when passing, or put on a table within easy reach of someone who loves to fiddle, who is restlessly up and down, or who sits still for a large amount of time.

- A personal rummage kit can be made around someone's memories – objects should trigger particular stories that can be retold. Include labels with notes on either aimed at the user – 'Remember using this dibber when you worked in the nursery?' – or at a staff member who works with the resident. Labels might include questions or trigger words, or a story that is familiar and can be fed back to the resident if they are no longer able to start it for themselves. This type of kit might be kept to one side and only used in reminiscence work with the resident for whom it is made. Try to find relevant items that work through all five senses – a CD of the factory whistle, a bottle of a favourite scent or fabric from a wedding dress. Whatever the contents, they must be personal – but so might the container be! What about a hat box, a vintage suitcase, an old fashioned biscuit tin?

- Theme kits are also a good idea – why not put together a 'Day at the sea' kit, with postcards, shells, sticks of rock, sunglasses and hats, sound effects and seaside songs, seaweed (great as a sensory smell as well as texture!), bucket and spade, then play 'We're all going to the seaside', unpacking the bag together, dressing up, and exploring the shells! The perfect 20-minute holiday where the weather doesn't matter! Also suit the container to the theme – a beach hold-all for the seaside, a box covered in cut-out snowflakes for a winter kit, a box wrapped in birthday paper for a party kit, or a tool box for a 'wee workie' kit!

- Create sensory kits for work with people in the later stages of dementia – look at the sensory profile I created for myself in the

'Sensory Activity' chapter earlier in the book (page 47). A kit for me might therefore contain grapefruit hand cream, pieces of leather, suede and fur, a bag of candyfloss, some chocolate and a CD of my favourite music and sounds.

- When I run theme days I often invest in a selection of costume accessories – a French Day was berets, neckerchiefs, stripy tops and plastic onions; a 'Pink Day' raising money for a cancer charity included wigs, sunglasses and witches hats. I am in the process of compiling one for National Talk Like a Pirate Day! Indulge in stereotypes! Give people what they expect to see, the 'idea that springs to mind', rather than trying to be accurate. Each fancy dress kit is then stored in a simple drawstring bag, the fabric matched to the event so that the contents are easy to identify, and reused as a dressing-up activity. The bags hang on pegs on the wall so I can grab one and go. I often include CDs, pictures, books, etc., so that we can dress up to music, or a story or a poem.

Sensory

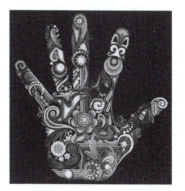

Some suggestions

- Sensory sessions can be the basis for one-on-one sessions, but can also work well in a group, or as part of another activity.

- Stimulate all the five senses – touch, taste, sight, hearing and smell.

- We have already looked at the way musical memory is stored separately to other types of memory. The same is true of smell – scents can act as a shortcut to memories that may otherwise be forgotten. Use smells to start a reminiscence session, or during cooking. Use them to stimulate or to relax. Run a smell quiz using the objects, or use talking about smells as a springboard to further discussion and reminiscence.

- Explore the sensations created by touching different textiles and items. One lady loves a chenille scarf and keeps it on her lap. She has very little speech, but the first time it was given to her she sat stroking it, looked up and said 'cat'.

- Hide objects in a bag and ask people to guess what they are touching.

- Explore human touch – remember that the centre of Tom Kitwood's flower was 'love' (see page 23). This is often expressed through touch – stroke or massage someone's hands, brush or stroke their hair, allow hugs to happen – the shoulder squeeze, the bear hug and the lean. Touch can feel threatening, however, so make sure you watch the resident for clues about whether this is okay – ask for permission if you are unsure. Remember that how comfortable someone feels can change day by day and moment by moment.

- Use a 'Guess that sound' CD, or different types of music or spoken word. Talk about the words themselves – most people have favourite words and language is fascinating.

- Run a tasting session with themed food or drink; how about different kinds of bread or fruit? The choice of even these basic foods can often be very limited in Care, so go crazy!

- Do some sensory cooking (see page 82) – the end product doesn't matter so long as everyone gets to try the ingredients by taste or smell, to lick the bowl and their fingers, and generally get messy and sticky...

- Blow bubbles – let others blow bubbles! But be aware that bubbles bursting on the skin can feel disturbing if you can't see them coming.

- Blow up balloons and play group or one-on-one balloon games.

- Be happy to play, and be guided by what works with a resident or a group of residents.

- Use dolls or teddy bears if this is appropriate for your residents. Don't underestimate the amount of comfort and love this can give.

- Enjoy the experience of using play dough – even if your modelling skills are poor, squidge it between your fingers. Did anyone else paint their hands with PVA glue at school and spend hours engrossed in peeling it off again?

- Play catch with bath puffs or flashing balls – use them in the bath instead of (or as well as) rubber ducks.

- Use scented lotions for hand (or foot) massage. NB: The use of aromatherapy oils must be checked with nursing staff as some can cause bad reactions.

- Run a nail care session. Wash hands in warm water with liquid soap. Collect all trimmings, etc. and dispose of quickly, sterilising nail clippers between residents. Use a gentle scented hand cream to massage hands. Allow residents to choose any nail polish colour – be complimentary! Work regularly so that chipped polish is removed in a day or two, and be prepared to take the polish off for anyone if it seems to be distressing them. Don't be afraid to offer a manicure to the gents! You don't have to use polish. NB: Polish contains various chemicals that may cause allergic reactions. If a client begins to have problems breathing or complains of a headache *stop* what you are doing, make sure there is lots of fresh air and contact nursing staff. Make sure you do not leave polish out unattended. Never cut toenails.

- Look at cheap projection items – there are various ones on the market that light the room with stars on the walls and ceiling, or are voice or music sensitive. Invest in a white umbrella and create a mini sensory experience for a resident, sit close together cocooned inside the umbrella's arch and use a coloured torch to project onto its canvas.

- Use wind chimes, rainbow wind spinners and plants with a nice smell, taste or texture, and create a sensory garden, even if it's only in one raised bed or on a window sill (see the Resources section at the end of this book).

- Put food out for the birds and watch them come to eat it. Put a CD with birdsong on.

- Hang a crystal in the window to make rainbows as the sun catches it. Or use a rainbow maker.

- Think about using senses that are undamaged – for a person who struggles to see, describe pictures or give them something to touch; give picture clues to someone who can't hear music, or help them to feel the vibrations.

- Bring fresh flowers in and let the residents enjoy the scent. Get them to touch the petals and leaves. They could make a display to share. When the flowers fade, pull the petals off and use them for a flower petal massage – pour them like confetti over someone's hands and crush them to release the smell. Use paper confetti if flowers are impractical.

- Bring chocolate buttons with you – just the right size to slip between the lips with the minimum of effort, and to melt on the tongue...

Spiritual and Religious

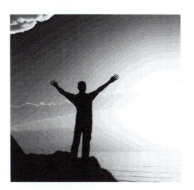

Spirituality and Religion
Risks

- It's easy to get bogged down in the idea that spirituality is the same as religion. Don't make this mistake! Everyone has spirituality – but not everyone has religion.

- People may become very emotional when dealing with spiritual needs. They may have been emotionally very badly damaged, and may have to work through things. Try not to be afraid, just be with them, and don't try to have all the answers.

- Our spiritual journey may not have anything in common with our residents' journeys, and it can be harder to remain objective. Again, try to just be with them, without judging.

- Don't make generalisations.

- Candles can be really useful props – although they may cause problems. Find out what your Home's policy is. We have been allowed tea lights for spiritual occasions if they are monitored by a member of staff (or spiritual celebrant) and never left alone.

Spirituality
Some suggestions

- Spirituality is *very* individual! Take a moment to think about what is important to you when you are not at work. Think about all the things you enjoy, the times, places, events or people that make you feel like the man in the picture above. It may be meditating with crystals, camping alone in the woods, reading, working in the garden, or being pampered at the local beauty parlour. Try to identify the feeling that this gives you. You may feel lit up, taller, as if you can breathe, full of energy, calm, at peace, connected.

- You will have to do some detective work to find out about what gives your residents these feelings. Many residents may be able to tell you, but for some you will need to work on a life story, and talk to family and friends. You may need to experiment with different possible answers – or accept that there are several answers. And some of the answers can be quite strange. One lady I know actually feels that part of her spirituality is having a good grumble and getting everything off her chest – she describes it as 'bleeding the radiators'!

- Discovering where people get their spiritual connection from will probably help you to work out what resources might be useful. A constant supply of chocolate or a pot of bubbles, some crystals or a candle should be easy to source.

- Finding out what makes someone tick can cause more problems, however – how do you meet the needs of someone who used to go off camping alone in the woods for a week at a time? What elements of that can you give back to them? It might be time outside (whatever the weather), or time alone. You might be able to source a CD of forest sounds, or something that smells like tent canvas and wet earth.

- Hold hands. Share time.

- Listen to music together.

- Laugh till it hurts!

- Eat chocolate.

- Make something together.

- Watch children playing, or hold a baby. You may need to borrow these...

- Talk about things that are worrying, or that are important to an individual.

- Make a Japanese wish tree – tie coloured ribbons to a tree, or a branch in a pot. Write wishes on coloured paper and tie these to the tree as well. If it's outside, or near a fan, the breeze will make the colours dance.

- Give someone a hug.

Religion
Some suggestions

- For many people, especially those from older generations, a spiritual connection is found through religion. A book of different world faiths may help you grasp the basic concepts and rules for various religions you may encounter. You can also find information on the internet.

- It is important that you find out how a person experienced/ experiences their religion – don't assume that Catholics don't eat fish on Friday, or that a Jew will always keep her hair covered. There is as much variety in how faith is practised as there is in anything else. Someone may greatly appreciate contact with a minister of their religion, and the chance to attend services. Or they may still identify themselves as, for example, a Christian, but may no longer be practising. As with any religious practice it is important for people to be able to continue to make connections and to follow important rituals. Some people may even be discovering religion for the first time.

- Try learning a prayer that is important and sharing it with an individual.

- Read or recite familiar passages together, such as the Lord's Prayer or Psalm 23 for a Christian, the Al-Fatiha for Muslims, the Shema for a Jew, the Sarvodaya for a Hindu or the Japji Sahib for Sikhs. Most religions use set language in services, so repetition over the years will mean that this is an enduring memory. Check out the relevant books in the Resources section at the end of this book, or even better, search for the prayers on YouTube – especially if there is no way you could recite these prayers yourself. There are videos of most of the prayers chanted by an imam or cantor.

- Try to make contact with local places of worship; see if they would be prepared to visit members of their congregation or faith in the Home, or to make recordings of parts of services for you to use.

- Contact your nearest cathedral – most have vast educational resources, both for Christianity and for other religions, which they lend out to schools and other establishments.

- A notable exception to structured western religion is Quakerism. Although it came out of the Christian tradition, it does not use Christian words and phrases, and considers itself separate. Quaker worship and spiritual journey is through sitting together in silence, with the occasional thought shared. Quakers hold the dying 'in the light', and a funeral can be a very joyous occasion.

- Celebrate religious occasions so that everyone can join in, regardless of faith. We recently celebrated the birthday of Krishna, a Hindu festival, in our very English middle-class Christian Home. Because we had no emotional involvement to the festival as a Hindu would, we explored the concept of divine love (Krishna is the god of divine love, among other things), and ended up talking about why we valued and loved one another – an incredibly moving experience, especially for those who considered themselves worthless now that they were disabled in some way.

- You may find that a minister or church visitor (of any religion) knows nothing about dementia, and may not understand why his or her congregation behaves in the way it does. You may have to share your understanding of the people you work with, and of how this might affect the service.

- Think about asking for a service to be adapted so that it becomes more 'dementia friendly'. Watching residents who come each time to a service, I noticed that some parts of the service seemed familiar to everyone. We've talked above about the repetition of prayer becoming an enduring memory – what about taking away everything that doesn't seem to have endured? Is it a problem if a Christian church celebration becomes the lighting of candles, the singing of familiar hymns and the saying together of the 'Lord's Prayer'? Does it matter if every service doesn't include communion? Only your residents can give you the answer to this, and ultimately it must be their wishes that are put first. Sadly, however, many of those visiting a Home will find it very hard to change. It may be that you need to ask several different temples or churches to all have input into services, and to run several different styles of worship, each geared to a slightly different group of residents.

- Another cause of strife may be that residents are experiencing dementia at different stages and with different expressions. Some may be perfectly able to be part of a traditional service, and to sit quietly in contemplation if the actual words and actions get away from them. Others may need prompting and guidance to do the same, but obviously find the experience meaningful. Try not to be afraid of offering this guidance, even though it may mean talking during the quiet bits, or bearing with someone who sings a different hymn to everyone else. Again this may be a cue for offering different types of service to different groups.

- It is also useful to be aware of the practicalities involved in giving services to people with dementia – instead of rice paper wafers for communion, which stick to damp lips, don't really look like something to eat and are not easy to swallow, and wine that can be a shock to a system unused to alcohol, and cause coughing, consider using a roll of bread torn and shared, and some red fruit drink.

My own background is Christian, and this is the type of service I can write about with confidence; it is also the type of service I have seen used in Care Homes most often. Each religion will come with its own challenges, however, and only by experiencing services with our residents can we see what might need to be changed.

Theme Days

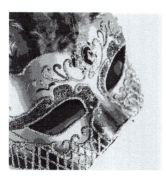

Suggested resources

The enthusiasm of at least one other person – this is not something you can do alone

Time and forward planning

Risks

- The day you plan may not appeal to people, or may be too hard to pull off at that moment.

- Lack of involvement from others can mean you are left on your own trying to do everything.

Some suggestions

- Think about who the day is for – I plan days that will appeal to staff or to residents or both at once. The staff I have worked with love to dress up, so a Pyjama Day to raise money for charity appeals to them – be aware that the residents may enjoy watching others make fools of themselves without wanting to be involved.

- Think about why you are doing the day – is it to raise money, as above, or to learn about a culture, religion or an event, or is it to celebrate something meaningful to your residents (the Royal Wedding), or to encourage staff and resident bonding (an African Day run by Zambian staff)? Is it a National Day with lots of resources available, or something only you will be doing?

- Try looking at the 'National Days of…' calendar online, or a religious calendar. We've celebrated everything from Talk Like a Pirate Day to Rosh Hashanah and St Piran's Day. Look online for resources for events.

- Get residents involved in planning or preparing for the day with craftwork, baking or decorating the space.

- Think about what day you will hold the event – do you want friends and family to join in, especially young children? Think about the time as well – early evening may be great for residents but it is really hard for families travelling from work or school.

- Make sure you advertise well – aim to get posters up at least one weekend before the event, hopefully catching the eye of visiting families. Include the date, time and location, as well as any dressing-up or attendance requirements.

- Think about the wording of posters – I used the phrases 'Wear your pyjamas all day' and 'Pyjama party' rather than 'Wear your pyjamas to work' – after all, the residents live in the Home, they don't work there.

- When planning your day try to get other departments involved – see if the chef will join you in planning a different menu. If menus are set, can you think up imaginative names for the dishes? Put a menu on the tables?

- Try moving dining room furniture around to give a different feel for the function.

- Think of a dressing-up theme and, if the budget allows, make sure you have accessories on hand to allow everyone to feel like they are part of things.

- Encourage staff to be involved, even if that means coming in on their day off.

- Run events just aimed at staff to boost morale and team spirit – I invite a local rep to run a chocolate party before Easter and Christmas that is particularly aimed at staff – although residents are never excluded from events (see www.chocolate-parties. com).

- Try to plan things that will appeal to both your very able residents and your sensory residents – include music, scents, spectating, tastes and accessories for tactile interest. Plan an event just aimed at one group or another – then balance things out with something else for others.

- Leave yourself time to clear up, enlisting residents where possible.

- Don't be over-ambitious – shorter or quieter events may work best for your group. A theme week may be easier for people to cope with – a trip to a destination on day one, a meal on day two, a concert or event on day three and a craft project or reminiscence event on day four may be less overwhelming than trying to do all of that in one day!

- Enlist the help of staff with particular talents or members of the local community. Talk to regular entertainers to see if they will enter into the spirit of an event. A musician who visits regularly was thrilled to dress up as a pirate and play sea shanties for us!

- Always consult with management before or during planning something, and try to make sure you debrief afterwards – check out what people think went well, or badly, and how such an event could be improved.

- Always thank people for their involvement. Making sure you say 'thank you', or providing an individual 'thank you' poster or a gift for someone who put a lot in, means that everyone feels much more like joining in again next time.

- Always have a camera, and make sure it's charged and has film or space in the memory. Take lots of photographs and make sure you display them so that everyone can relive the event!

Talk Like a Pirate Day

Why? Well, why not?! This was a day I felt could appeal to staff and residents. I started planning some weeks in advance – I experimented with different ways I could structure the day, and different ideas I could incorporate.

Talk Like a Pirate Day

WHAT DO I WANT TO INCLUDE?

- Dressing-up for staff – get hold of accessories for residents to dress up?
- Music – sensory appeal.
- Silly games? Children's party feel? Plan to include grandchildren.
- Treasure Island – advance craft project? Gold coins, buried treasure.
- Fishing game? Is this 'piratical' enough?? Cannonballs? Balloons?
- Decorate dining room? Table centres, palm trees?
- All day? Party idea, just afternoon?
- Food or drink? Pirates, grog/rum? Tea trolley themed? Doctor menu?

ADVANCE PLAN

- Saturday afternoon event encouraging families and staff with children.
- Live music important – contact musician and ask about dates – as near Sept 17th as poss.
- Discuss dates with management and confirm, tell Heads of Dept, book dining room.

- Talk to chef re menus and tea trolley.

- Advance activity sessions: poster making, paint Treasure Island game.

- Discuss with management and head of care about staff dressing up.

- Contact local fancy dress shop about hiring accessories and what we could get for our money. What can we make or borrow for free? Hats, bandanas, patches, parrots, hooks? Waistcoats, boots, wigs, cutlasses?

- Buy gold coins for prize.

- Re-use table centres from Jamaica Day.

- Make sure posters go up two weeks in advance to generate interest.

PLAN FOR THE DAY

- Pirate menus and dining room decorations put up during am. Involve able residents. Blow up balloons, get camera, name badges and pens ready.

- Musician arrives at 2pm. Assist residents to dining room, seats set up for cannonball game.

- Musician to play whilst dressing-up articles handed out, staff encouraged to sit with residents, children encouraged to help dish out.

- Remembering to 'talk like a pirate', introduce the cannon ball game – opposite sides of dining room into two teams – suggestions for names of ships. Equal numbers of balloons to each team. Whilst music plays send all cannon balls to opposing team – dirty tactics allowed! End of game fewest balloons in your 'ship' win.

- Posing for photos – one staff member to work with camera and musician to take piratical photos, second staff member to ask people to suggest pirate name – name badges written and dished out. Encourage spectating of photos.

- Use treasure map to 'dig for buried treasure' – pick a grid square, note next to name. Musician to open envelope with solution, treasure to be awarded.

- Tea trolley with high tea cakes, scones, etc. (resident choice), staff to enjoy with residents.

- Singing to finish afternoon.

- Thank everyone involved!

AFTER THE EVENT

- Develop photos, make 'thank you' posters for individuals, display photos on notice board.

- Talk about the day with staff and residents – what went well? What didn't people enjoy? Informal chats only.

- Send thank you to musician.

- Return any hired or borrowed outfits.

Ramadan and Krishna Janmashtami

This was part of a year of festivals aimed at finding out about other religions and traditions, as well as celebrating those already dear to our hearts. Ramadan was aimed at the more sensory residents I worked with at the time, Krishna Janmashtami at the more able. I discovered early on that it is not possible to get excited about celebrating a festival you know nothing about, and have no connection to, so the interest had to come from what we did.

Ramadan
WHAT DO I WANT TO INCLUDE?

- Sensory level, so food and music, tactile experiences, doing and exploring.

- Gentle event, peaceful, slow pace, not too many things in short time.

- More able residents will still choose to come along, so something for them to enjoy as well, but not focused on them. Give info about religion.

- Run up events – craftwork? Wall hanging? Art and architecture?

- Look at websites for what is important to this festival – fasting, food, purification.

ADVANCE PLAN

- Midweek event, afternoon session. Cooking involved so check with chef. Book room.

- Advance crafts – use source pictures from internet to create laminated table mats – involve more able residents. Spend time looking at source pictures, exploring shapes and colours with more sensory residents. Wall hanging – ladies craft group involved in creating – collage, not sewing. Exploring fabrics, textures, etc. Use sewing skills – cutting paper patterns, pinning to fabric to cut out, etc. Involve others in sorting buttons, use to create texture and interest. Simple painted border. Encourage staff to drop in and help.

- Select recipes – authentic, but easy to use in care environment. One very simple, one more complex. Lots of different things to taste/smell. Buy ingredients.

- Source appropriate CD of music.

PLAN FOR THE DAY

- Wall hanging and table mats out during morning.

- After lunch put CD on and gather residents.

- Fade out music to aid concentration. Bring bowl and warm water, spend time with each resident washing hands – talk about purification, use scented soap.

- Look at the wall hanging – take people close so they can explore the textures and colours.

- Talk about fasting, and how important special food is to celebrations. Divide group; one staff member to work with more able residents (or put very able resident in charge) on date cake – make sure everyone in both groups gets to taste and smell ingredients. In more sensory group make mint lemonade – enjoy the shape and smell of lemons before cut. Get everyone to smell lemons, work together to squeeze juice. Have sugar in bowl so easy to access – spoon into mix. Enjoy fizz of water bottle opening, and sound of pouring – get people to help with each stage. Everyone to stir, taste – enough sugar? Share mint leaves, crush to smell, allow people to eat if wanted. Tear up and add to lemonade. Taste. When cake is cooked, bring to group to share cutting, smell of new cake, eat with fingers to feel warm crumbly texture.
- Remember to take pictures!
- Thank everyone for coming and put CD on for a few minutes before people start to leave.

AFTER THE EVENT
- Develop and display pictures, make 'thank you' posters.
- Observe participants and make notes of what went well or was enjoyed, and what might need to be done differently.
- Consider running the session again with a closed group of more sensory clients, or on a different unit. What other events or recipes might work in this format?

Krishna Janmashtami
WHAT DO I WANT TO INCLUDE?
- Primarily for more able residents, but to include sensory residents as well.
- In-house day, no outside entertainers, midweek.
- Look at difference between religions with single god and multiple gods. Similarities between religions – Krishna inspires divine love between his followers, joy and caring

for one another. Opportunity to discuss feeling hopeless and useless in care (theme has been very present in overheard conversations in last weeks)?

- Particular dance associated with festival – Rasa Lal – stick dance – can we incorporate something like this? What internet resources are there that would support this? Include appropriate music.

- Get able residents to share info? Things to read out? Make this interesting? Beetle drive? Single-step game that gives info to share?

- Where can I get hold of objects to share and explore? Diocese Resource Centre?

ADVANCE PLAN

- Look at internet resources for Rasa Lal dance – YouTube videos. Choreograph simple moves that can be done seated or standing!

- Contact Resource Centre and book any resources they may have available.

- Source pictures of Hindu gods and their attributes for beetle drive game. Make up myself so that info is new at time of playing.

- Advance craft: use sticks left over from May Day and decorate with ribbons for Rasa Lal dance. Lots of tactile and colour exploration with ribbons.

- Find dice for beetle drive – prizes?

- Collect resources from Resource Centre.

PLAN FOR THE DAY

- Set up shrine with object from Resource Centre during am – available to explore during day.

- Gather labels, felt-tip pens, plain paper, beetle drive equipment, CD player and music, brightly coloured fabrics to decorate tables.

- Set up room with chairs grouped round small tables draped in fabrics. All chairs need to have good view of shrine. Use sliding coffee tables so that they can be easily removed later.

- Welcome everyone with CD of background music playing.

- Explain about Hindu religion, brightness and colour, excitement. One god with many attributes, each with their own name and personality. Explore objects in shrine.

- Play beetle drive – each card will have a god on one side, and info about him/her on the back. Award prizes to winners, ask member of each team to read info about their deity. Play again, shifting round cards. Introduce Krishna in last round.

- Krishna's birthday; his attribute is not just making mischief, but love of those around us. Talk about what each person values most about themselves, and what the group as a whole value about this person. Write on labels and give to each person. Keep a note for later. Spend time as needed talking about these values, about how hard it can be sometimes to remember the positives.

- Wake the mood up again – music for dance – demonstrate! Hand out sticks, go through movements, try with music! Give it several goes, calling pattern as needed. Congratulate everyone! Reward with cups of tea!

- Mention that this week's film will contain a version of this dance so they should all come and watch it!

- Thank everyone for taking part; encourage them to keep their labels.

AFTER THE EVENT

- Use the notes made about what we value to make up individual posters for people to keep; include some source pics, e.g. a stick dance, and Krishna.

- Watch participants and chat as appropriate as to how they felt about the session. Has the overall mood lifted?

- Is there a need for more sessions like this? Is this something I can do? What help might I need?

Trips Out

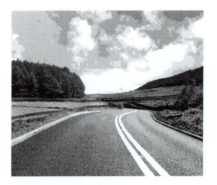

Suggested resources

Courage!   Picnic basket

Contact details of the local dial-a-
ride scheme, bus/minibus hire (look
for companies with tail lifts), or a
bus of your own! (Dare to dream!)

Risks

- Exhaustion or over-excitement!

- Losing someone – always count out and in, and make sure you
  have sufficient staff to support the particular residents you are
  taking.

- Losing *things* – from handbags to false teeth… If you are getting
  out of the bus make sure you are aware of personal possessions.
  If the bus windows are open, think who you sit next to them!

- Vomiting! Make sure you take bowls, bags, gloves and wipes. Try to find out from families about travel sickness in a person's past. Think about using anti-sickness pills before leaving for anyone who may suffer. Take sucking sweets, like barley sugar, to give out during the journey.

- Personal injury. Risk-assess for likely problems and have strategies in place for coping. You should take at least one first aider and a first aid kit.

- Make sure the bus has valid breakdown cover.

- If you are planning to be out for a long time, make sure you take any appropriate medication or continence products.

- Always take a charged mobile phone that has been topped up.

Some suggestions

- Start small! Try walks in the garden to see how people respond to being out of their usual environment.

- Talk to management. There are more potential problems to this kind of activity than any other, as you are separated from the usual support team. If something goes wrong, you – and your manager – need to feel confident that you can handle it.

- It depends greatly on your role as to what kind of trip it would be appropriate for you to run. If you have no experience or training you will need to make suggestions to management, but be led by their decisions. You will also need to persuade other staff that this is a good idea, as you will not be able to do this alone. If you are part of an activities team you will still need to be guided by management, but may have more success getting the ball rolling. Much depends on the individual Home.

- If you are planning a trip in a hired bus, talk to the company and explain briefly about the needs of your residents. It may be that they are frail and that you need a tail lift as they can't do stairs; it may be that you want to take residents who can't transfer from a wheelchair to a seat and need to find out about wheelchair spaces. It may also be that your residents are in the later stages of dementia and may do things that, to people who don't know them, seem odd. You may also need to explain some of your staff for similar reasons! A colleague of mine is prone to demanding we stop suddenly – it's usually because she's seen something she wants to share with residents (like a man trout fishing), but if you have no warning, she can be quite alarming!

- If using your own bus, make sure you have enough fuel, or money to buy some.

- Really think about who you are taking and what kind of trip might work for them. You should be getting to know people well by now, and if you are not sure, talk to other staff. I find that often the length of a trip is dictated by how far along someone is in their dementia. I offer short trips more frequently to later-stage residents, and longer trips to those who are more able. You need to feel confident in running a trip, but residents coming on it need to feel confident too! Build positive memories, and soon you will find you have a waiting list!

- I recently had a carer placed with the activities team for a short while. She was amazed at how different it was to be out with residents in our bus. She noticed that people were more animated, that they noticed and chatted about the scenery and weather; they started to share memories and stories. A lady who seemed incapable of any decision was suddenly certain about the fact that she wanted coffee to drink, thank you! People forgot about their weak bladders and didn't need the toilet once when we were out for three hours. Someone who regularly refused food would accept cake and a drink. 'We get to be friends – not us and them!' she commented when we came back.

- Consider 'comfort breaks', and if you are not going to have any then warn residents on their first trip. They will soon be able to judge for themselves whether they can manage. Make sure that anyone who needs it is wearing a continence pad, and take spares if you think it may be necessary. Also think about getting back in time so that everyone can go to the toilet comfortably before the next meal.

- Favourite short trips for our residents include coffee at a local supermarket cafe or at the garden centre, parking by the canal and watching the boats, going up to a local view point, driving along the river, or even just looping out through town and back.

- Medium-length trips include taking the picnic basket with tea, coffee and biscuits, and parking on a village green under the trees, or by a river, exploring favourite routes through the local countryside, going 'scrumping' for apples in the autumn, collecting conkers (horse chestnuts) or photographing spring flowers for a display.

- Longer or more challenging trips include a day at the seaside, visiting the local theatre that is half an hour away, the carol concert for one of our link schools 45 minutes away, going round the cathedral, Christmas shopping, visiting the sailing club (no, we didn't actually go sailing...) and a pub lunch.

- We find that taking our residents to a place full of other people can be really challenging. If you are used to living with a small group of people, where every day is predictable, and your memory is not going to be challenged in a big way, going to a large event full of other people can mean system overload. Negotiate with your local theatre group and see if they will let you attend dress rehearsals instead of going to a full performance. Go to the flower show at the local church the day after it finishes (by arrangement, don't just turn up!). People can be wonderfully kind about helping you to make someone's day!

- If people are struggling to stay oriented during a trip try giving them a memory card. I took a gentleman to concerts and noticed that he would suddenly look stressed, and find it hard to settle. I started writing on his programme where we were, who he was with, and what time we would go back to the Care Home. He would read the information, check I was there, check his watch, and then settle back again. Sometimes he would check that information every two minutes, but as long as it worked, I kept taking him.

- Be aware that a severe stroke may leave a person with little or no body feedback. Trips may be intensely frightening as they become lost in space with no feeling of their body sitting securely belted into a seat.

- Welcome relatives on trips. They will often give a real care boost, and it may mean they get some really good time with their relative. One gent used to come with his wife and us to the local supermarket; they would go off and do their own thing, then meet us to come home. It made all the difference to their continued relationship. But do think about practicalities – it is no good if the relative becomes one more person who needs looking after. Talk things through with your team members.

- Cancel trips if you do not feel safe, for example if the weather is really bad, or if you do not have enough support.

- If you are trying to get regular trips started, make sure you write down who went, where you went, and all the positive feedback you got. Also write down what didn't go so well and possible solutions – and whether *they* worked.

Afterword

Once upon a time, there was a wise man who used to go to the ocean to do his writing. He had a habit of walking on the beach before he began his work.

One day, as he was walking along the shore, he looked down the beach and saw a human figure moving like a dancer. He smiled to himself at the thought of someone who would dance to the day, and so, he walked faster to catch up.

As he got closer, he noticed that the figure was that of a young man, and that what he was doing was not dancing at all. The young man was reaching down to the shore, picking up small objects, and throwing them into the ocean.

The wise man came closer still and called out, 'Good morning! May I ask what it is that you are doing?'

The young man paused, looked up, and replied, 'Throwing starfish into the ocean.'

'I must ask, then, why are you throwing starfish into the ocean?' asked the somewhat startled wise man.

To this, the young man replied, 'The sun is up and the tide is going out. If I don't throw them in, they'll die.'

Upon hearing this, the wise man commented, 'But, young man, do you not realise that there are miles and miles of beach and there are starfish all along every mile? You can't possibly make a difference!'

At this, the young man bent down, picked up yet another starfish, and threw it into the ocean. As it met the water, he said, 'It made a difference for that one.'

Adapted from 'The Star Thrower' by Loren Eiseley (1969)

Some days it seems hopeless. So many people and so many needs. One person cannot meet them all, cannot change everything, cannot fix it all. One person can only be there for one person. Just one. And then another one. And another. We meet needs by constantly adding drops to the ocean. This is real life, and it isn't perfect. We just do the best we can. Remember, 'It made a difference for that one.'

Resources

Part I

Dementia

www.alzheimers.org.uk – home of the UK's Alzheimer's Society, with information for those with a diagnosis and their caregivers. Look out for details of local Alzheimer's cafes and 'Singing for the Brain' groups that you could join with your residents. The Society also runs a gay carers helpline.

www.alz.org – Alzheimer's Association in the US; their education and resource centre.

www.ageuk.org.uk – Age Concern and Help the Aged joined to become Age UK.

www.dementiafoundation.org.au – Dementia Foundation, Australia, 'trying to create a different future for dementia'.

www.dementiacareaustralia.com – Dementia Care Australia.

www.dementiaknowledgebroker.ca – Canadian dementia resource and knowledge exchange.

www.alzheimer.ca – this site has an interesting 'quiz' about attitudes to those with dementia.

www.dementiacarematters.com – offers David M. Sheard's view of dementia care; there is a very good video of him explaining his philosophy. Most training is corporate, but there is a page of articles to download which gives lots of insights and ideas.

UK Journal of Dementia Care – covers all sorts of different strands of dementia care, and consistently includes articles on activities. (Subscription for individuals is expensive so try to persuade your manager to subscribe for the Home.)

Dementia Reconsidered: The Person Comes First (Rethinking Ageing) by Tom Kitwood (Open University Press, 1997).

Understanding Alzheimer's Disease & Other Dementias by Dr Nori Graham and Dr James Warner (Family Doctor Publications, 2009). This is one in a series of books created for local chemists to sell; it is jargon free, giving accurate and accessible information. It has been recommended by Barbara Pointon, MBE.

www.memorybridge.org – a groundbreaking documentary that reveals the largely unrecognised capacity of people with Alzheimer's and related dementias.

Assessing

The Pool Activity Level (PAL) Instrument for Occupational Profiling: A Practical Resource for Carers of People with Cognitive Impairment (Bradford Dementia Group Good Practice Guides) by Jackie Pool (Jessica Kingsley Publishers, 2007).

Care to Communicate: Helping the Older Person with Dementia by Jennie Powell and Eve Morris (Hawker Publications, 2000).

www.theactivitydirectorsoffice.com – Activity Director Today, an Australian one-stop shop which includes such marvels as templates for assessment documents, etc.

Life story

www.lifestorynetwork.org.uk – includes clips showing filmmaking and animation as life story work.

www.knowmewell.com – downloadable publishing tool for professional printed books can be found here.

www.lifebio.com – helps people create an autobiography or the biography of a loved one by using LifeBio's carefully crafted questions or by using their Memory Journal or other reminiscence products.

www.forgetmenotbook.com – a UK-based company who created a life story tool online. Customers sign up on behalf of a loved one, invite friends and family to contribute stories and photographs to the site by logging on, and they can then order printed books full of the stories and pictures. Post is worldwide and prices are in both pounds and dollars. The layout of the book is limited to make it easy for anyone to use.

www.ageuk.org.uk/health-wellbeing/relationships-and-family/older-lesbian-gay-and-bisexual – lesbian, gay, bisexual and transgender section of Age UK's site.

www.ageuk.org.uk/Documents/EN-GB/Information-guides/AgeUKIG02_Lesbian_gay_or_bisexual_inf.pdf?dtrk=true – 'Lesbian, Gay or Bisexual: Planning for Later Life' booklet.

Living at Home with Alzheimer's Disease and Related Dementias: A Manual of Resources, References and Information by Carol Bowlby Sifton (Canadian Association of Occupational Therapists in partnership with Alzheimer Society of Canada, 1998).

Planning

The Activity Year Book: A Week by Week Guide for Use in Elderly Day and Residential Care by Anni Bowden and Nancy Lewthwaite (Jessica Kingsley Publishers, 2009), a week-by-week activity guide for one year, with a theme per week, games quizzes and exercises to fit each theme.

Joining in

www.napa-activities.co.uk – NAPA publishes lots of booklets aimed at showing all staff that they are part of the activity cycle.

Recording

www.photo.jessops.com – the Jessops Photo Printing site has one of the easiest book tools to use.

www.snapfish.com/snapfish/aboutUs – look at the bottom of the page for links to its country-specific sites.

www.shutterfly.com – US-based, but ships worldwide.

www.bonusprint.com – for photo books, etc.

www.blurb.com – make your own book site.

www.extrafilm.com.au – Australian site for making your own books.

www.photobookamerica.com – US site.

www.acilab.com – American Color Imaging.

Sensory activity

The Calm Technique: The Easy Way to Beat Stress Instantly Through Simple Meditation Methods by Paul Wilson (Thorsons, 1997).

Environment and reality orientation

'Chatter Matters' is available from Colin Barnes at colin.barnes@solent.nhs.uk.

Contented Dementia: 24-hour Wraparound Care for Lifelong Well-being by Oliver James (Vermillion, 2009) explains Penny Garner's SPECAL (Specialised Early Care for Alzheimer's) method of dementia care.

Using activity to 'solve problems'

And Still the Music Plays: Stories of People with Dementia by Graham Stokes (Hawker Publications, 2010).

Budgeting

www.better-fundraising-ideas.com – fundraising ideas.

Money Raising Activities for Community Groups: A 'Funds and Fun' Guide for Agency and Community Fairs, Bazaars, and Other Money Raising Events by Virginia W. Musselman (Association Press) was first published in 1969, but despite that, it still has some good ideas for events, and for making them run smoothly.

Training

www.napa-activities.co.uk – runs an accredited level 2 activities distance learning course, as well as specialist day courses through the Red Cross.

www.orchardtrusttraining.co.uk – runs level 2 and level 3 activity provision courses from their centre in the Forest of Dean.

www.dementiauk.org – runs day courses in London on a variety of subjects. They also offer bespoke training in Care Homes.

www.nccap.org – the National Certification Council for Activity Professionals (NCCAP) is a US organisation that certifies activity professionals who work with older people. Various levels of certification are available, and all work can be done online, so overseas enrolment is a possibility.

www.activitydirector.net – American site that has online activities courses and resources.

www.dementiacafe.com – offers various dementia training courses. They also have other information available on their site.

www.careprofessionals.org – American training site focused on dementia.

www.u-first.ca – Canadian site with online training modules in dementia care.

General

The Good Practice Guide to Therapeutic Activities with Older People in Care Settings by Tessa Perrin (Speechmark Publishing, 2005) – a brilliant book from NAPA that provides a benchmark against which we can measure and evaluate our practice. It has links to national standards, provides guidance for Care Home owners and managers wanting to set up activities, and calls for clinical governance in the emerging 'profession' of activity provision.

Keeping Busy: A Handbook of Activities for Persons with Dementia by James R. Dowling (The Johns Hopkins University Press, 1995) – an entire book of word games, exercises and activities used by a Care Home in the US.

How to Make Your Care Home Fun: Simple Activities for People of All Abilities by Kenneth Agar (Jessica Kingsley Publishers, 2008) – written by a Care Quality Commission inspector and member of the Alzheimer's Society, this book has some great ideas and will give you background information on the legal aspects of running a Care Home.

Alzheimer's Activities That Stimulate the Mind by Emilia Bazan-Salazar (McGraw-Hill Professional, 2005) – a very American take on activities, mainly aimed at those caring for a loved one at home, this book has some useful input, although it can be overly technical and believes strongly in reality orientation.

www.elderlyactivities.co.uk – created by The Consortium Care, it has downloadable doable activities, or you can upload your own suggestions.

www.elder-one-stop.com – an American site with suggestions on activity and living in old age.

www.speechmark.net – a shop of resources which also produces a monthly e-zine; see www.elderlyresources.co.uk for more details.

www.scie.org.uk – Social Care Institute for Excellence online care resource full of short films about best practice.

www.age-exchange.org.uk – a leading UK charity working in the field of reminiscence.

www.agedcarer.com.au – provides online articles for Australians caring for ageing relatives.

www.nscchealth.nsw.gov.au/carersupport/carersupportprojects – Northern Sydney Central Coast health website.

www.agedcareguide.com.au – DPS guide.

www.fightdementia.org.au – lots of information and support for caregivers as well as those with a diagnosis, online shop, courses, fact sheets and more.

www.dementiasupport.com.au – as above, with some very interesting courses on offer.

www.savvysenior.org – amazing American signposting site with links to everything from fitness, pensions and government support to the National Senior Games and online dating sites.

www.best-alzheimers-products.com – exciting American site with lots of different types of product available.

www.alz.uci.edu – American Institute for Memory Impairments and Neurological Disorders, with lots of interesting videos about life and research.

www.alzinfo.org – Fisher Center for Alzheimer's research.

www.nia.nih.gov/alzheimers – America's National Institute on Ageing educational and referral centre.

www.myhomelife.org.uk – promotes quality of life for those living, dying, visiting and working in Care Homes.

www.baringfoundation.org.uk – provides downloadable reports on the value of the arts in elderly and residential care.

Part II
Art
The Expressive Arts Activity Book: A Resource for Professionals by Suzanne Darley, Wende Heath and Mark Darley (illustrator) (Jessica Kingsley Publishers, 2007) – an amazing and insightful book about using art to make connections.

Activities for Older People: A Practical Workbook of Art and Craft Projects by Brian W. Banks (Butterworth-Heinemann, 2000) – based on the author's own experience, this book is packed full of workable art and craft ideas.

Art Therapy Exercises: Inspirational and Practical Ideas to Stimulate the Imagination by Liesl Silverstone (Jessica Kingsley Publishers, 2009) – tried-and-tested exercises.

www.veilpainting.wordpress.com – this and the following two sites are examples of veil painting – www.lovingcolor.org/id14.html and www.philosophyoffreedom.com/fgallery/283.

Books

The Reader Organisation have produced a book called *A Little, Aloud*, comprised of pieces of prose and poetry picked around a theme with notes about how others have responded to the pieces. The organisation also run training, but it's expensive. Contact them on 0151 794 2830 or www.thereader.org.uk.

I would recommend the *Nations Favourite* books, selections of favourite comic or love poems, hymns or general poetry. The contents seem to be immediately familiar to many people.

www.alzpoetry.com – dedicated to using poetry with those with a dementia. Provides suggestions, books, training and so forth.

www.picturestoshare.co.uk – enables you to create books of beautiful pictures around various themes.

www.flora.org/homeschool-ca/resources.html#menu – Canadian resource aimed at home schooling families, but has lots of further links to all sorts of further resources, from 'Mail a tale' to publishers of specialist resources.

Shakespeare: The Animated Tales, edited by Leon Garfield (Heinemann Young Books, 1998).

Cooking

'Good Housekeeping': Successful Microwave Baking by the Good Housekeeping Institute (Ebury Press, 1987).

For supplies, see:

> www.lakeland.co.uk
>
> www.bakewaredirect.com.au
>
> www.alibaba.com/showroom/silicone-bakeware.html
>
> www.siliconemoulds.com
>
> www.canadiantire.ca

Crafts

www.scrapstoresuk.org – a charity that runs stores selling clean, reusable scrap to schools, Care Homes and other organisations, as well as discounted art and craft supplies. They have branches across the UK.

www.artshape.co.uk – a Gloucestershire-based charity that runs workshops, sells 'art in a box' products, etc., available through their enquiry form.

www.bakerross.co.uk – craft products and ideas online or via a catalogue at reasonable prices.

www.riotstores.com.au – Australian craft store chain with materials to buy and suggestions on what to make.

www.eckersleys.com.au – similar to the above, selling goods to both individuals and organisations.

www.michaels.com – American and Canadian online and real time arts and crafts store with suggestions of projects to make.

www.deserres.ca – similar to the above, based in Canada.

Exercise

www.vitalyz.co.uk – exercise equipment, resources and training. Was very impressed that the training included how to create a version of their equipment from cheap goods!

www.petsastherapy.org – supplies volunteer animals and their owners to visit Care Homes, covered by their own insurance. You can register interest online, or contact a local placement officer.

www.recsport.sa.gov.au – offers downloadable posters aimed at keeping the over-50s age group active, and runs training on how to support this group during physical activity.

www.helpguide.org/life/workouts_exercise_overweight_disabled. htm – has some really good suggestions and links for further information around starting and continuing an exercise programme.

www.amazon.com/Seniors-Exercise-DVD-Osteoporosis-Alzheimers/dp/B0007MVXRK – an American series of DVDs (region 1) for elder exercise.

www.flaghouse.com – Canadian physical equipment store.

Working with Elderly People by Anne Murphy (Souvenir Press Ltd, 1994) contains a chapter of easy seated exercises that can be done to music, complete with amusing diagrams.

Exercise for Frail Elders by Elizabeth Best-Martini and Kim A. Botenhagen-DiGenova (Human Kinetics Publishers, 2003) is full of background technical information, what to do and what not to do, checklists, etc., as well as a series of workout programmes with photographs of real older people undertaking the exercises.

Armchair Exercises for Fitness Phobics: Everyday Maintenance for the Busy, Tired, Elderly, Infirm, and Straightforward Lazy by Sue Hooker and Maggie Humphry (Trafford Publishing, 2007) – I've yet to try this one with my residents, but it looks fun.

Rosie's Armchair Exercises: A Complete Body Workout from the Comfort of Your Own Armchair by Rosita Evans (Discovery Books, 2011) – a small book with a surprisingly challenging workout which is do-able in an armchair or wheelchair, although please exercise caution!

Games

PT Games Ltd, PO Box 74, Newcastle Upon Tyne, NE99 1BL, Tel. 0191 274 8101 – provides a range of games that are dispatched on a sale or return basis. Sensible prices.

The Finishing Lines by Beckie Karras (ElderSong Publications, 2008) – includes proverb quizzes, quotes and advice.

Gardening

Design for Nature in Dementia Care by Garuth Chalfont (Jessica Kingsley Publishers, 2007) – okay, so you can't redesign your Home, or (probably) the garden, but there are lots of other suggestions for bringing nature to residents.

www.livingleavescare.co.uk – creates therapy gardens for Care Homes. They are pricey, but they are happy to offer advice, and have a show garden in Hampshire which you can visit.

www.thrive.org.uk – runs training and sells publications around gardening for those with a disability.

www.abc.net.au/gardening/stories/s3621525.htm – a wonderful video and write-up about a sensory garden in an aged care facility in Melbourne, Australia.

The following sites offer food for thought on what you might try to include in a sensory garden, be it a small pot, or 'a series of gardens dedicated to the senses':

www.motherearthliving.com/gardening/sensory-garden-lawrence-kansas.aspx

www.bbc.co.uk/gardening/gardening_with_children/plantstotry_sensory.shtml

www.leevalley.com – Canadian site with a range of gardening resources.

The following sites have ideas for feeding garden birds with fat balls:

www.wildaboutanimals.forumotion.net/t651-fat-ball-cake-recipe-for-birds

www.instructables.com/id/How-to-make-fat-ball-bird-feeders/?ALLSTEPS

Knitting

Crochet Unravelled: A Clear and Concise Guide to Learning Crochet by Claire Bojczuk (Pottage Publishing, 2005).

Granny-Square Crochet – 35 Contemporary Projects Using Traditional Techniques by Catherine Hirst (CICO Books, 2012).

Granny Square Love: A New Twist on a Crochet Classic for Your Home by Sarah London (F&W, 2011).

Granny Squares: Over 25 Creative Ways to Crochet the Classic Pattern by Stephanie Gohr, Melanie Sturm and Barbara Wilder (Search Press, 2012).

Knit a Square/Make a Toy (Home Library Craftbooks) (Cole Publishing Company, 2000).

Knitty Gritty: Knitting for the Absolute Beginner by Aneeta Patel (A & C Black Publishers, 2008).

Music

www.3choirs.org – runs Mindsong that creates music therapy opportunities for people with dementia, as well as training in running music groups and in circle dancing.

www.pastperfect.com – specialises in CDs of various 'vintage' music from the 1920s on.

www.memorylane.org.uk – a UK-based 'radio' station that creates half-hour programmes fully saveable to your computer of dance music from the 1920s, 1930s and 1940s. They also make and sell CDs and DVDs as well as producing a regular newsletter for subscribers.

www.shopercussion.ca – a Canadian percussion instrument site that is probably beyond the budget of most of us, although it has interesting facts about the history and playing methods of different types of percussion, which I found very interesting.

www.lpmusic.com – an American site which is rather more affordable than the above; it has a series of video tutorials on different types of percussion.

www.nordoff-robbins.org.uk – a music charity.

http://steinhardt.nyu.edu/music/nordoff – Steinhardt School of Culture, Education and Human Development, based in New York.

www.nordoff-robbins.com.au – another link to the Nordoff Robbins Music Therapy Foundation, with information on what they do, courses and ways to get involved.

www.musictherapy.org – American Music Therapy Association.

www.stmarysmusic.org – link for recordings of first verses of hymns; the link is not live yet so in order to access it, contact the choir master (director@stmarysmusic.org).

Group Music Activities for Adults with Intellectual and Developmental Disabilities by Maria Ramey (Jessica Kingsley Publishers, 2011) – complete with CD, although it does recommend other music.

Melody Lingers On: A Complete Music Activities Program for Older Adults by Bill Messenger (Venture Publishing, 2004) – currently out of print, but it does come up on Amazon as second-hand quite often. Very American, but lots of the songs are common to both UK and American cultures. Includes a CD, exercise programme, sing-a-longs, quizzes and anecdotes about the music.

The Ulverscroft Large Print Song Book by Glyn Lehmann and Margaret Donald (F.A. Thorpe, 1987) – provides a range of well-known songs to sing along to in either a music edition arranged for piano with guitar chords, or a large print words-only edition.

Say it With Music: Music Games and Trivia by Beckie Karras (ElderSong Publications, 1990) – offers a range of quizzes from 'Complete the song title' to 'Guess the instrument'.

Reminiscence
Remembering Yesterday, Caring Today: Reminiscence in Dementia Care: A Guide to Good Practice by Pam Schweitzer (Jessica Kingsley Publishers, 2008).

www.europeanreminiscencenetwork.org – set up by Pam Schweitzer, the network runs training and projects in the UK, US, Australia and Canada, as well as many other countries.

www.manyhappyreturns.org – picture cards and training for reminiscence.

www.vintageradio.org.uk – radio by and for the over-50s. Based in Merseyside, it broadcasts across the country via this internet link.

www.fiftiesweb.com – 1950s reminiscence site.

www.dailysparkle.co.uk – a daily or weekly downloadable reminiscence newspaper for residents.

www.alzheimersproducts.blogspot.co.uk – all sorts of products available to purchase, with a particular emphasis on reminiscence photographs from the UK, US and Australia.

www.age-exchange.org.uk/projects/past/mappingmemories – suggestions and guidance for reminiscence with minority ethnic elders. Generally this site is great and has lots to offer!

www.winslowresources.com – produces packs of photo cards around different topics for reminiscence.

Sensory

www.exploreyoursenses.co.uk, www.cheapdisabilityaids.co.uk and www.sensorytoywarehouse.com – voice-activated mood lights, projectors, etc. at reasonable prices.

Pifco Star Master – projects stars onto the walls and ceiling. Static or colour change programmes.

www.home2garden.co.uk – wind chimes and spinners. See also:

www.windcreations.co.uk

www.windchimescorner.co.uk

www.sensorytoywarehouse.com – has an adults and elderly section, and will ship worldwide.

www.specialneedstoys.com – has stores in a variety of countries, including the UK, US and Canada.

www.tecsol.com.au – sensory equipment, but pricey.

For two videos and a series of articles about the use of dolls as therapy, see:

www.youtube.com/watch?v=Pp8aKaWN7EI and www.youtube.com/watch?v=1X1zPVI4fZE

www.dementiacareaustralia.com/index.php?option=com_content&task=view&id=60&Itemid=81

www.dementiadoctor.co.uk/dolltherapy.html

www.medicalnewstoday.com/releases/223519.php

www.best-alzheimers-products.com/doll-therapy-for-alzheimers-disease.html

www.voices.yahoo.com/doll-therapy-alzheimers-disease-1836626.html

Spiritual and religious

Person Centred Counselling for People with Dementia: Making Sense of Self by Danuta Lipinska (Jessica Kingsley Publishers, 2009).

The Methodist Homes Association and the Christian Council on Ageing produce booklets and literature around religion and spirituality, not just with a Christian bias. See www.mha.org.uk and www.ccoa.org.uk for information. For example, *Religious Practice and People with Dementia* explores the five main faiths in Britain at the moment and includes the prayers mentioned in the main text. All the literature is very reasonably priced.

Worshipping with Dementia: Meditations, Scriptures and Prayers by Louise Morse (Monarch Books, 2010) – gives mini services that can be delivered on a one-on-one or small group basis with familiar readings and scripture.

www.presencecareproject.com – looks at living with dementia from a spiritual angle, particularly the technique of mindfulness. Based in the US, the website posts regular short articles and stories about the people they meet daily. They also run training.

www.niichro.com/cfc/cfc_6.html – a Canadian site focused on Inuit and Indian groups and their needs.

www.stmarysmusic.org – link for recording of first verses of hymns; the link is not live yet so in order to access it, contact the choir master (director@stmarysmusic.org).

www.stpancraschurch.org – a London church that 'takes ageing and Spirituality seriously' – enjoy their resources.

General resources

www.activitiestoshare.co.uk – a rapidly expanding specialist product resource. Prices vary, but many items are affordable.

www.activitiesforcarehomes.co.uk – a range of products and activity suggestions with a free monthly quiz to which you can subscribe.

www.outwoodcare.co.uk – a growing range of life skills packs and furniture; unfortunately prices are high.

www.ageappropriateresources.co.uk – an interesting range of resources for the exercise of both mind and body – as well as for having fun!

www.winslowresources.com – provides a wide range of publications and activity resources including music, quizzes and so forth from their own publishing house.

www.alzstore.com – provides up-to-date products and resources to guide people in their journeys with Alzheimer's and dementia.

www.sablier.com – Canadian company specialising in equipment, reminiscence and resources for seniors.

www.education.spectrum-nasco.ca – Canadian educational resources company with wide range of special educational needs resources.

www.carersuk.org, www.carersaustralia.com.au and http://caregivers.vch.ca/resources_web.htm (signposting to support for caregivers) – don't forget, you need support too!

Index